MW01221879

Retinoids

Retinoids

A Clinician's Guide

Second Edition

Edited by

Nicholas J. Lowe, MD, FRCP, FACP
Clinical Professor of Medicine and Dermatology, UCLA School of Medicine, Los Angeles
Director, Southern California Dermatology and Psoriasis Center, Santa Monica, California, USA
and Cranley Clinic, London, England

and

Ronald Marks, BSc, FRCP, FRCPath
Professor of Dermatology, University of Wales College of Medicine

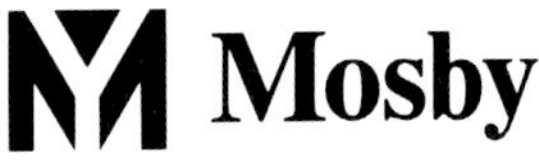

St. Louis Baltimore Boston Carlsbad Chicago Naples New York Philadelphia Portland
London Madrid Mexico City Singapore Sydney Tokyo Toronto Wiesbaden

Although every effort has been made to ensure that drug doses and other information are presented accurately in this publication, the ultimate responsibility rests with the prescribing physician. Neither the publishers nor the authors can be held responsible for errors or for any consequences arising from the use of information contained herein.

First published in the United Kingdom in 1995 by
Martin Dunitz Ltd
The Livery House
7–9 Pratt Street
London NW1 0AE

Second edition 1998

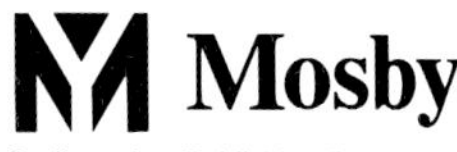

A Times Mirror Company

Distributed in the U.S.A. and Canada by

Mosby–Year Book
11830 Westline Industrial Drive
St. Louis, Missouri 63146

Times Mirror Professional Publishing Ltd.
130 Flaska Drive
Markham, Ontario L6G 1B8

A CIP catalogue record for this book is available from the British Library

ISBN 1 85317 427 0

Composition by Scribe Design, Gillingham, Kent

Printed and bound in Spain by Grafos, S.A. Arte sobre papel

Contents

List of contributors

Roshantha Chandraratna, PhD, MBA is at Allergan, Irvine, California, USA.

Michael J. Connor, PhD is at the Division of Dermatology, UCLA School of Medicine, Los Angeles, USA.

Michael David, MD is Head of the Department of Dermatology, Beilinson Medical Center, Sackler School of Medicine, Tel Aviv University, Israel.

Elliott Klein, PhD is at the Department of Biological Sciences, Allergan, Irvine, California, USA.

Nicholas Lowe, MD, FRCP, FACP is Clinical Professor of Medicine and Dermatology at the UCLA School of Medicine, Los Angeles, and Director of the Southern California Dermatology and Psoriasis Center, Santa Monica, California, USA and Cranley Clinic, London, England

Ronald Marks, BSc, FRCP, FRCPath is Professor of Dermatology at the University of Wales College of Medicine, Cardiff, UK.

Ola Rollman, MD, PhD is at the Department of Dermatology, University Hospital, Uppsala, Sweden.

Braham Shroot, PhD is Vice-General Director of the Centre International de Recherches Dermatologiques, Galderma, Valbonne, France.

Anders Vahlquist, MD, PhD is Clinical Professor at the Department of Dermatology, University Hospital, Uppsala, Sweden.

Introduction

The last 25 years have seen increasing use of synthetic retinoids for a variety of skin disorders. It seems that the dermatologists of the 1940s and 1950s may have been right – vitamin A does have rather special actions on the skin.

Topical retinoids remain amongst the most widely used treatments for selected types of acne. They are particularly effective in treating the superficial varieties of this disorder characterized by small papules and comedones. More recently, the new topical retinoids, tazarotene and adapalene, have been shown to be effective in acne.

Tazarotene is likely to be a significant advance for topical psoriasis therapy. It is, in effect, the first topically effective retinoid for psoriasis.

In recent years the action of topical tretinoin and isotretinoin on photodamaged skin has made a major impact on dermatology. The next decade will bring other clinical uses for topical retinoids as well as novel retinoid agents which may be effective topically.

Systemic retinoids have been shown to be highly effective in a number of different diseases. Isotretinoin continues to be indicated for therapy of severe nodulocystic acne and acne that is poorly responsive to conventional therapy. Isotretinoin has revolutionized the treatment of these severe forms of acne. However, as with other systemic retinoids, it has important side–effects and careful patient education and instruction are needed prior to its use. It is a teratogen and it is therefore important that women of childbearing potential are not treated if there is any risk of becoming pregnant during or shortly after treatment.

Etretinate has been available for almost a decade for the treatment of severe forms of psoriasis and other disorders of keratinization. As a result of the storage problem and prolonged excretion of etretinate, the carboxylic acid derivative known as acitretin has now been developed. While this is more rapidly and completely excreted than etretinate, there have been concerns that small amounts of this drug may be esterified to an etretinate–like metabolite in the presence of alcohol. It is therefore important that fertile women are cautioned to avoid pregnancy during therapy with acitretin, in the same way that they are for etretinate, for up to 1 or 2 years after discontinuation of the drug. Acitretin is now available in many countries worldwide and is gradually replacing etretinate. They are effective as monotherapy for plaque psoriasis, and most effectively used in combination with other forms of treatment, including ultraviolet phototherapy. It is worthwhile emphasizing again that both these drugs should only be used with extreme caution in fertile women because of potentially teratogenic levels remaining in the body for some years after discontinuation of the drug. Effective contraceptive measures are vital for this group.

The severe disorders of keratinization are rare but cause considerable disability. They too are much helped by the oral retinoid drugs. Patients with multiple skin cancers may also be helped by the retinoid drugs – both topical and systemic.

Apart from their acknowledged teratogenicity, the systemic retinoids have a wide range of toxic side–effects. Essentially these are of two types – common and trivial but aggravating, and uncommon and potentially serious. These are discussed in detail in this volume but it is worth noting here that the more serious side–effects include hyperlipidaemia, skeletal toxicity and hepatoxicity. It is a tribute to the unique efficacies of these drugs that despite their potentially significant side–effects they are extensively used and widely appreciated. There is little doubt in the minds of both the prescribing dermatologist and the patient for whom they are prescribed that the oral retinoids 'do things' that nothing else can. They are surely a very major milestone in the history of the development of treatments for skin disorder.

Our purpose in this book is to review the use of the retinoid drugs in clinical practice, paying particular attention to new developments in topical retinoid therapy, and the practical aspects of the subject. We sincerely hope that the book will provide guidance for the practising dermatologist.

1 Mechanisms of retinoid action in the skin

Michael J Connor

Introduction

The therapeutic use of retinoids has had an exciting and revolutionary impact on dermatology. The discovery of their efficacy in the curative treatment of previously recalcitrant cystic acne was probably the most significant advance in the treatment of skin disease since the introduction of corticosteroids. Again, as with corticosteroids, retinoids have proved useful in the treatment of a host of dermatological complaints. New applications may emerge as newer compounds are formulated. The aim of this chapter is to address the questions of how and why retinoids are so useful in the general dermatological arsenal.

Cutaneous retinoid metabolism

The term 'retinoid' applies to both the naturally occurring forms of vitamin A and the many thousands of synthetic analogues that mimic some of the chemical or biological activities of vitamin A. Although it has been recognized for many years that vitamin A itself has an important role in the maintenance and functioning of epithelial tissues, it is only recently that we have seen the emergence of hard evidence describing the potential molecular mechanisms involved in their biological activities.

Perhaps because synthetic retinoids are usually screened for activity in assays responsive to vitamin A-like structures, the clinically significant retinoids developed to date act as vitamin A agonists. It therefore seems likely that the therapeutically effective synthetic retinoids work through similar mechanisms to those of the physiological congeners of vitamin A. The value of retinoids as dermatological agents highlights the need for an understanding of these mechanisms of action in cutaneous tissues.

Although several minor metabolites have been detected, retinoic acid isomers are now clearly established as the most important vitamin A congeners in the skin. The major forms of vitamin A found within the cell are fatty acid esters of retinol, which are generally viewed as a storage form for retinol. Retinoic acid is synthesized within cutaneous tissues in two distinct steps from retinol: retinol to retinaldehyde (retinal), and retinaldehyde to retinoic acid.[1] Treatment of mouse skin with citral (3,7-dimethyl-2,6-octadienal), which inhibits both steps leading to retinoic acid synthesis,[2] also inhibits the biological activity of retinol in epidermis,[3] underlining the importance of this metabolic route. The molecular basis for the biological activity of retinoic acid isomers has been established to be mediated largely through two series of nuclear retinoic acid receptors. These receptors contain DNA-binding domains, and can directly regulate the expression of several gene products.

Retinoids show poor solubility in water and a propensity to bind non-specifically to hydrophobic binding sites. Circulating and cellular retinoids are therefore usually found associated with a carrier protein. Retinol is transported in the blood attached to serum retinol-binding protein (sRBP). Retinoids within the cells are shuttled around bound to low-molecular-weight binding proteins, principally forms of cellular retinol-binding proteins (CRBP) or cellular retinoic acid-binding proteins (CRABP). Although their importance in retinoid action has been eclipsed somewhat by the discovery of the retinoic acid receptors, these proteins play a role in mediating some facets of retinoid action, including the presentation of retinol to metabolizing enzymes and possibly acting as sinks to regulate cellular retinoid levels.

A major route for the inactivation of retinol and retinoic acid appears to be via cytochrome P450-mediated hydroxylation. The drug liarozole is a P450 inhibitor. Its moderate anti-psoriatic activity has been attributed to its ability to block the degradation of retinoic acid and thus enhance endogenous cellular retinoic acid levels.[4]

Molecular basis for retinoid action

The two groups of nuclear retinoic acid receptor proteins are members of the steroid hormone receptor 'superfamily'. They are dealt with extensively elsewhere in this book, and are treated only briefly here. The first group to be discovered, the RAR (retinoic acid receptor) group includes three major forms: RAR-α, RAR-β and RAR-γ. The skin is particularly rich in RAR-γ. These three proteins utilize all-*trans*-retinoic acid as their natural substrate. The second group, the RXR family (for retinoid-X (i.e. unknown) receptor) appear to utilize the 9-*cis*-retinoic acid isomer as the natural ligand. In general terms, genes that contain a RARE (retinoic acid response element) sequence in their promoter region can be activated by the nuclear retinoid receptors. Functional proteins of the steroid hormone receptor superfamily are dimeric, but their monomers have the ability to dimerize with monomers of related proteins within the superfamily to form heterodimers. The many different possible heterodimer combinations allow a considerable variation in both ligand binding and gene activation. The RXR proteins can form heterodimers that do not require their retinoic acid ligand for activation. This potentially enormous variation may explain the molecular basis for the range of activities shown by retinoid analogues and differences in response between tissues. It is also of great therapeutic significance. If different biological effects of retinoids are mediated through different receptors, it may be possible to develop clinically useful retinoids with minimal side-effects.

To date, the bulk of genes with RAREs expressed in skin that have been identified have proved to be concerned with aspects of retinoid metabolism or handling, including CRABP II, CRBP and RAR-β itself. Perhaps this is not too surprising, since it has long been known that levels of enzymes involved in retinoid metabolism are sensitive to vitamin A status. What is evident is that control of intracellular retinoid homeostasis is a complex and carefully regulated process.

Cutaneous effects of retinoids

The answer to the question of why retinoids are so useful in such a variety of skin disorders lies in their potent impact on almost all cutaneous structures. Cell, tissue and clinical studies have repeatedly demonstrated the ability of retinoids to modify the architecture of the epidermis, dermis and sebaceous glands directly. Systemic effects such as immunopotentiation[5] may also contribute to their efficacy.

Because the response of skin cells grown in culture has generally failed to mimic responses seen in vivo, emphasis is placed here on whole animal or clinical human studies. Most experimental studies of retinoid action have involved manipulation of tissue levels either by dietary deprivation or through supplementation, since these are the most convenient conditions to arrange experimentally. The paradigm for early investigations is the classic histological study of Wolbach and Howe,[6] who studied nutritionally deprived rats. While this and other early studies are problematic in that the diets used were poorly defined by today's standards and were probably deficient in a number of essential factors besides vitamin A, Wolbach and Howe observed in deprived rats that major changes occurred in the mucosal epithelia—a metaplastic transformation from a mucosal to a keratinizing epithelium—but noted that there was little or no change in skin histology. Because the skin is a keratinizing and not a mucosal epithelium, the lack of such a metaplastic change is not surprising. Later, clinical observations of follicular abnormalities in humans fed poor or restricted diets that responded to vitamin A therapy indicated an important cutaneous role for vitamin A, and perhaps foreshadowed the later therapeutic use of retinoids in the treatment of acne.

In the 1940s, with the isolation, determination and synthesis of vitamin A, investigators turned to investigating the impact of supplementation. Although conducted prior to the discovery of the importance of vitamin A metabolites, most of the cutaneous responses and changes that are now considered important facets of their activity were established early on. Most of this work was conducted with rodents, particularly strains of mice, and such studies have continued to the present. Because rodents are hirsute, investigators used either non-glabrous skin (the ears and tail) or utilized one of the hairless mutant strains that have been available since the late nineteenth century. Three areas are of particular relevance: studies of the impact of retinoids on the ultrastructure and biochemistry of 'normal' hairless mice; studies of 'rhino' mice (their abnormal follicular structure has lead to their advocation as a model for acne, and the ability of vitamin A derivatives to correct the pronounced wrinkling of their skin presaged the use of retinoids in addressing skin ageing); and studies of the differential effects of retinoids on rodent tail skin ultrastructure (their scaly tail skin includes parakeratotic regions reminiscent of psoriasis).

Typical histological responses to acute and chronic local application of retinoids to hairless mouse[7] or human skin[8] include hyperproliferation leading to a dose-dependent expansion of the numbers of cell layers of the stratum spinosum and stratum granulosum, but (provided the dose is subtoxic) with little change in the number of cell layers of the stratum corneum. The basal cells may appear more elongated than usual—an appearance more typical of basal cells in hyperproliferative states—but the number of basal cells per unit length and the number of basal cell layers are unchanged. The hyperplasia occurs in both the interfollicular and the contiguous follicular epidermis. Retinoids also induce epidermal hyperplasia in mice after systemic administration, although higher dosage levels are needed to achieve delivery of sufficient retinoid to the epidermis.

In murine models the dose range inducing a dose-dependent hyperplastic response is such that toxicity, if it does occur, is usually limited to mild scaling. This occurs at retinoid doses below those inducing other cutaneous symptoms of toxicity, and is a sensitive indicator that higher doses will be toxic. In contrast to the appearance of the epidermis after low to moderate doses of retinoids, moderate to severely toxic doses may result in a decrease in the stratum granulosum, a thinning of the interfollicular epidermis, some acantholysis, erythema and general tissue fragility.[9] In severe cases, epidermal erosion and subcorneal pustules form under a parakeratotic stratum corneum, and the sebocytes may become granular and lose lipid. This contrasts with the almost-normal appearance of the sebaceous glands seen after lower concentrations of retinoids. Recent studies have clearly established that this toxicity is mediated by RARs and is not some non-specific irritant response. RAR-γ is the major nuclear receptor found in mouse epidermis. Engineered mice with a disrupted RAR-γ gene showed a marked resistance to retinoid-induced toxicity.[10] Treatment with AGN 193109, an RAR antagonist, considerably reduced the toxicity associated with treatment with toxic doses of retinoic acid or the potent retinoid TTNPB.[11]

Since the number of epidermal cell layers reflects the equilibrium between cell formation and ultimate cell loss through desquamation, increased cell production provides a ready explanation for the induction of epidermal hyperplasia by retinoids. However, if retinoids inhibited epidermal desquamation or a late step in cell differentiation or maturation then the hyperplasia could partly reflect accumulation of incompletely differentiated or immature cells. In this respect, retinoic acid has been found to decrease 'cornified envelope'—a possible marker for keratinocyte terminal differentiation—in epidermal cells cultured in vitro under certain conditions. Results from our in vivo studies were incompatible with abnormal maturation because there was no change in the number of stratum corneum cell layers, nor was there evidence of any imbalance in the relative numbers of stratum granulosum and stratum spinosum cell layers following single or multiple retinoid treatments. Epidermal transglutaminase is localized in mouse epidermis to the stratum granulosum.[12] The localization was similar in retinoid-induced hyperplastic epidermis, but the band of straining was more marked and broader, reflecting the increased thickness of the stratum granulosum. The specific activity of the transglutaminase activity found in epidermal extracts was not changed by retinoid treatment, but the absolute amount (activity per unit area of skin surface) markedly increased with time to a maximum at 4–5 days, corresponding to the time of maximum epidermal hyperplasia. This difference in relative and absolute amounts reflects the retinoid-induced hyperplastic state, i.e. the net increase in the number of layers of differentiating cells per unit area of skin. The transglutaminase activity per unit that was found in epidermal extracts after various doses of all-*trans*-retinoic acid was directly proportional to the number of cell layers of the stratum granulosum. The individual cells of the stratum granulosum thus appear to express similar levels of transglutaminase in both unstimulated and retinoid-induced hyperplastic epidermis.[12] Stratum corneum turnover, measured by disappearance of fluorescence from dansyl chloride-stained skin, was more rapid in the retinoid-treated mice.[12] Since both the formation of epidermal cells and the loss of differentiated cells are increased by retinoid treatment, reduction of cell loss through inhibition of epidermal cell differentiation or delayed maturation does not account for the retinoid-induced hyperplasia. The hyperplasia is almost certainly a consequence of an increased production of cells that otherwise show the histological, biochemical and physiological behaviour of cells competent for normal differentiation.

The most striking feature of mature 'rhino' hairless mice is the gross rugosity (wrinkling) of their skin. Histologically, characteristic follicle-derived horn-filled rounded cysts are present in the epidermis and dermis. In 1949, Frazer[13] reported that chronic feeding of vitamin A esters to these animals prevented the development of the characteristic rugosity and stopped the progressive enlargement of some of the cysts. Later, Van Scott[14] reported that topically applied retinoic acid had a dramatic effect on the histology, restoring the upper follicles to a more normal-appearing structure, and Kligman and Kligman[15] confirmed that topical retinoic acid, as reported for systemic vitamin A, could reduce the rugosity.

Detailed histological studies reveal that topical retinoids induce a dose-dependent hyperplasia in both interfollicular and utricular epidermis and reduce utricle diameter.[9] The utricle walls thicken concomitant with a change in the shape of the utricles to that resembling the normal follicles of hairless mice. This 'redifferentiation' or 'remodelling' of the utricles to more normal-looking follicles occurred only at retinoid doses above those that induced epidermal hyperplasia for a variety of retinoids of different potencies. Follicular hyperplasia is often more evident near the base around the opening of the sebaceous glands. This differential response may be involved in the straightening of the otherwise rounded utricles. The response to higher toxic doses is clearly distinguished: the epidermal architecture is abnormal, the stratum granulosum is less evident, acantholysis may occur, and there is a marked shrinking and granularization of the sebaceous glands.[9] The histological data suggested that retinoids were enhancing production of differentiation-competent cells, and that this stimulation may be driving the changes in epidermal and follicular morphology. In a recent investigation using a series of RAR-γ-selective retinoids, an excellent correlation was found between efficacy in reducing rhino mouse utricules and toxicity assessed in the rabbit irritancy model,[16] indicating that both efficacy and toxicity are under RAR control in this system.

One of the more prominent defects in psoriasis is the absence of stratum granulosum from affected areas and the concomitant retention of nuclei in the overlying stratum corneum. The tail skin of rodents has regions of parakeratosis interspersed with orthokeratotic zones. The histological response of these parakeratotic regions was once commonly used as a bioassay for potential anti-psoriatic agents. Topical treatment with retinoids leads to dramatic changes in the parakeratotic regions.[17] Retinoids stimulate the appearance of a prominent granular cell layer, leading ultimately to a more orthokeratotic ultrastructure. It was this ability of retinoids to stimulate the differentiation process in parakeratotic regions in favour of orthokeratosis that led to their use in the therapy of psoriasis. Although results from early clinical intervention studies relying on use of natural retinoids were mixed, the success of the retinoic acid analogue etretin and its ester etretinate in ameliorating psoriasis has stimulated the development of more efficacious anti-psoriatic retinoids.

The anti-acne drug isotretinoin (Accutane, 13-*cis*-retinoic acid), is one of the most widely used retinoids in clinical practice. In common with many retinoids, it readily isomerizes in the presence of light to a variety of isomers, including all-*trans*-retinoic acid. Since topically applied all-*trans*-retinoic acid is useful in the therapy of mild acne, some of the therapeutic benefit of isotretinoin may be mediated by this route. However, systemic isotretinoin is far superior to all-*trans*-retinoic acid in the successful treatment of nodulocystic acne. In addition to exerting effects on the follicular epidermis similar to those seen with topical all-*trans*-retinoic acid, 13-*cis*-retinoic acid exhibits an unusual property in humans. After systemic administration of therapeutic doses, 13-*cis*-retinoic acid induces a dose-dependent reduction in sebum secretion from the sebaceous glands which has a pivotal role in its therapeutic action against severe cystic acne. A comparable response has yet to be observed after administration of other retinoids to humans, with the caveat that relatively few retinoids have been thoroughly evaluated in the systemic therapy of acne. Although a reduction in sebaceous gland size or activity has only been observed in the skin of animal models at severely toxic doses,[9] since retinoid toxicity is RAR mediated it would seem likely that the anti-sebic effect of 13-*cis*-retinoic acid in humans is similarly RAR mediated. Because topical application of 13-*cis*-retinoic acid is far less efficacious than systemic delivery, it is not clear if the anti-sebic action of 13-*cis*-retinoic acid is a direct effect of the retinoid on the sebaceous glands themselves, or if it is mediated by a systemically formed metabolite (although none has so far been identified). Additionally, 13-*cis*-retinoic acid functions as an immunopotentiator, that is, it stimulates antibody production against otherwise subliminal levels of an antigen in acne patients.[5]

Retinoids and skin cancer

Retinoids have shown potent antineoplastic effects against many malignant cell types. In many of these cases, the underlying mechanism is the triggering of terminal differentiation or the expression of a less malignant phenotype. Unfortunately, clinical and experimental studies of retinoids and skin carcinogenesis have produced mixed results to date. Locally applied retinoids have been reported both to enhance and to inhibit tumour promotion in multistage chemically induced skin cancer studies in mice. Similarly, retinoic acid has been reported to greatly enhance, inhibit or have no effect on UVB-induced skin carcinogenesis in mice.

Part of the answer to these contradictions lies in the complexity of the system underlying retinoid action. Although the skin is retinoid responsive, vitamin A deficiency itself has minimal impact on gross or microscopic epidermal morphology. However, vitamin A deficiency does have cutaneous effects. Skin-tumour promotion is inhibited in vitamin A-deficient mice.[18] Furthermore, tumour expression is vitamin A dependent, since tumours appeared when vitamin A-deficient mice were re-fed retinyl palmitate or the provitamin β-carotene. Citral, which inhibits retinoic acid formation, also inhibits tumour promotion.[19] These results suggest a physiological requirement for retinoids, particularly retinoic acid, for tumours to appear.

Although clinical use of retinoic acid as a topically applied anti-acne agent dates back more than 20 years, no studies have directly addressed associated changes in skin cancer rates in the treatment population. Clinical trials of retinoids as chemopreventives or as chemotherapeutics for established cancerous lesions have, as with the animal studies, produced mixed results. However, there is a growing body of data demonstrating the efficacy of topical all-*trans*-retinoic acid against low-grade possibly premalignant lesions such as actinic keratoses.

Retinoids and ageing skin

The efficacy of topical retinoic acid in the treatment of photodamaged skin and as an 'anti-wrinkle' agent, moderate though it may be, has led to much popular as well as scientific interest. However, the mechanism underlying its action is still unclear. While favourable changes in epidermal histology are evident, this does not explain the decrease in rugosity, since skin elasticity is clearly provided by the dermal connective tissue. Fisher et al[20] have proposed that retinoic acid functions in the dermis by reducing UVB induction of metalloproteinases, which can degrade dermal matrix proteins. This is achieved indirectly by RAR repression of the activity of AP-1 (activator protein 1), AP-1 being a stimulator of metalloproteinase induction. Further studies should help to strengthen this hypothesis.

References

1. Connor MJ, Smit MH, Retinoic acid formation from retinol in the skin. *Biochem Pharmacol* (1987) **36**: 919–24.
2. Connor MJ, Smit MH, Terminal group oxidation of retinol by mouse epidermis; inhibition in vitro and in vivo. *Biochem J* (1987) **244**: 489–92.
3. Connor MJ, Oxidation of retinol to retinoic acid as a requirement for biological activity in the epidermis. *Cancer Res* (1988) **48**: 7038–40.
4. Dockx P, Decree J, Degreef H, Inhibition of the metabolism of endogenous retinoic acid as treatment for severe psoriasis: an open study with oral liarozole. *Br J Dermatol* (1995) **133**: 426–32.
5. Sidell N, Connor MJ, Borok M, Lowe NJ, Effect of a systemic retinoid on immune responses to specific protein antigens in humans. *J Invest Dermatol* (1990) **95**: 597–602.
6. Wolbach SB, Howe PR, Tissue changes following deprivation of fat soluble vitamin A. *J Exp Med* (1925) **42**: 753–77.
7. Connor MJ, Ashton AR, Lowe NJ, A comparative study of the induction of epidermal hyperplasia by natural and synthetic retinoids. *J Pharmacol Exp Ther* (1986) **237**: 31–5.
8. Connor MJ, Epidermal responses to retinoids in vivo. In: Dawson MI, Okamura WH (eds), *The chemistry and biology of synthetic retinoids*. CRC Press: Boca Raton, FL, 1990, pp 485–99.
9. Ashton RE, Connor MJ, Lowe NJ, Histological changes in the skin of the rhino mouse induced by retinoids. *J Invest Dermatol* (1984) **82**: 632–5.
10. Look J, Landwehr J, Bauer F et al, Marked resistance of RAR gamma-deficient mice to the toxic effects of retinoic acid. *Am J Physiol* (1995) **269**: E91–8.
11. Standeven AM, Johnson AT, Escobar M, Chandaratna RA, Specific antagonist of retinoid toxicity in mice. *Toxicol Appl Pharmacol* (1996) **138**: 169–75.
12. Connor MJ, Retinoid stimulation of epidermal differentiation in vivo. *Life Sci* (1986) **38**: 1807–12.
13. Frazer FC, The effect of vitamin A on hereditary hyperkeratosis in the mouse. *Can J Res* (1949) **27**: 179.
14. Van Scott JE, Experimental animal integumental models for screening potential dermatologic drugs. *Advances in Biology of Skin* (1972) **12**: 523–33.
15. Kligman LH, Kligman AM, The effect on rhino mouse skin of agents which influence keratinization and exfoliation. *J Invest Dermatol* (1979) **73**: 354–8.
16. Chen S, Ostrowski J, Whiting G et al, Retinoic acid receptor gamma mediates topical retinoid efficacy and irritation in animal models. *J Invest Dermatol* (1995) **104**: 779–83.
17. Jarrett A, Spearman R, Vitamin A and the skin. *Br J Dermatol* (1970) **82**: 197–9.
18. De Luca LM, Shores R, Spangler EF, Wenk M, Inhibition of initiator–promoter-induced skin tumorigenesis in female SENCAR mice fed a vitamin A deficient diet and reappearance of tumors in mice fed a diet adequate in retinoid or β-carotene. *Cancer Res* (1989) **49**: 5400–6.
19. Connor MJ, Modulation of skin tumor formation in mouse skin by the food additive citral (3,7-dimethyl-2,6-octadienal). *Cancer Lett* (1991) **56**: 25–8.
20. Fisher GJ, Datta SC, Talwar HS et al, Molecular basis of sun-induced premature skin ageing and retinoid antagonism. *Nature* (1996) **379**: 335–9.

2 Transport mechanisms and specific receptors

Braham Shroot

Introduction

The fine control mechanisms required to mediate cellular growth, differentiation and embryonic development are not yet fully understood. A major advance in this area of research has been made with the discovery that retinoic acid exerts hormone-like and morphogenetic effects. The initial recognition by McCollum and Davis[1] of a fat-soluble factor in certain foods, the demonstration of the role of vitamin A in vision[2] and the recent interest in putative anti-cancer action of β-carotene[3] underscore the major biological roles that these polyunsaturated lipophilic derivatives play. In this chapter we focus on how vitamin A and its derivatives are transported and act at the tissue, cellular and subcellular levels in the body. Special attention will be given to the skin in view of the extensive pharmacology which these substances manifest in this target organ.

Retinoid transport proteins and receptors

A generalized scheme for the generation of vitamin A and its derivatives from β-carotene has been proposed recently by Napoli and Race.[4] Essentially, it is postulated that, in the intestine, β-carotene is oxidized to retinol (vitamin A), which is in turn esterified to retinyl esters or oxidized to retinoic acid (RA). In the liver, stored retinyl esters can be hydrolysed back to retinol which binds to a plasma retinol-binding protein. This complex is then transported via the blood to target cells in which re-esterification and further oxidation can be effected (Figure 2.1). There is also evidence to support the idea that β-carotene may be directly transported from the intestine to the target cells where it may be converted to its active metabolites.[5]

Specific binding proteins

Plasma retinol-binding protein (RBP)

This is an extracellular protein (mol. mass 21 kDa) which specifically binds to retinol and has a high degree of sequence homology (about 70 per cent) within species. RBP binds with high affinity to another plasma protein transthyretin (TTR) as a one-to-one molar complex, which is sensitive to ionic strength

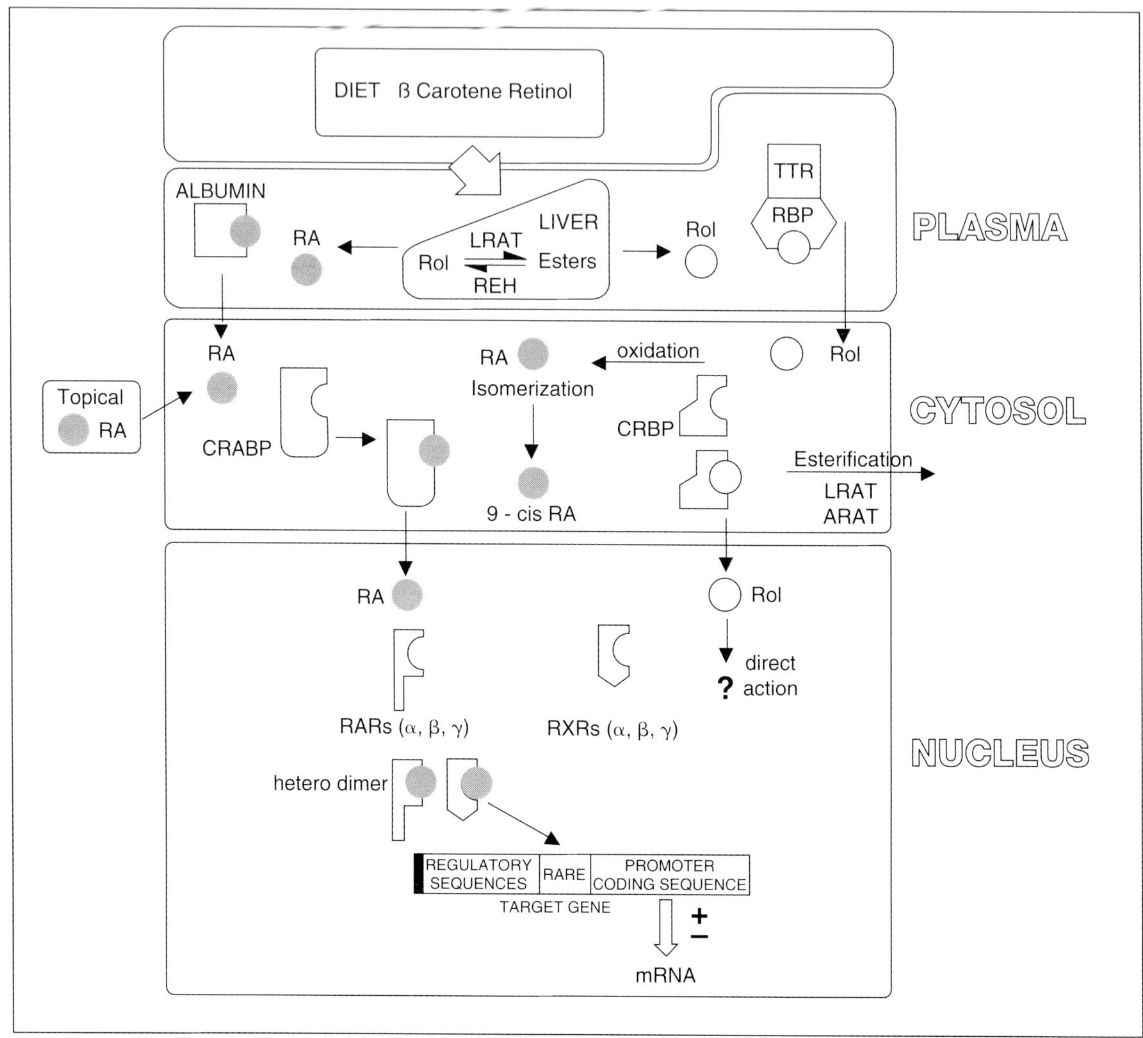

Figure 2.1

Generalized scheme for the generation of vitamin A and its derivatives from β-carotene.
RA, retinoic acid; Rol, retinol; TTR, transthyretin; RBP, retinol-binding protein; REH, retin ester hydrolase; LRAT, lecithin retinol acyl transferase; ARAT, acyl-CoA retinol transferase; CRBP, cellular retinol-binding proteins; CRABP, cytosolic retinoic acid-binding proteins; RAR, retinoic acid receptor; RARE, retinoic acid-responsive element.

and pH. The structure and expression of the RBP gene are well documented and it has been shown, using in situ hybridization techniques, that it is expressed in the liver, kidney and many other extrahepatic tissues. A detailed review has been published recently.[6]

Table 2.1 Binding properties of retinoids

Binding protein	*Source*	*Substrate*	K_d (M)	*Reference*
RBP	Rat testis	Retinol	8.9×10^{-8}	53
		Retinol	1.6×10^{-8}	55
RBP	Bovine serum	Retinol	7×10^{-8}	54
RBP	Rat insulinoma RINm5F	Retinol	8.6×10^{-9}	56
CRABP	Rat testis	RA	318×10^{-9}	53
		RA	$4.2\text{–}10^{-9}$	13
CRABP	Fetal hamster	RA	12.7×10^{-9}	58
CRABP	HL60	RA	1.5×10^{-9}	59
CRABP II	Neonatal rat skin	RA	6.5×10^{-8}	12
CRABP I	Human keratinocytes	RA	16.6×10^{-9}	60
CRABP II	Human keratinocytes	RA	50×10^{-9}	60
RAR-α	TRSF COS 1	RA	6.1×10^{-9}	57
RAR-β	TRSF COS 1	RA	7.6×10^{-9}	57
RAR-α	HBD *E.coli*	RA	6.2×10^{-9}	57
RAR-β	HBD *E.coli*	RA	8.0×10^{-9}	57

Cellular retinol-binding proteins (CRBPs)

This type of cellular protein is distributed in many organs,[7] has a molecular mass of 15 kDa and has a high affinity for all-*trans*-retinol ($\times 10^{-8}$M). Two CRBPs (CRBP I and II) binding retinol with high affinity have been characterized to date. These differ in their tissue distribution and in their pattern of expression during fetal and neonatal development.[8] In the rat, CRBP is mainly expressed in the liver, small intestines and testes, but an appreciable level is also found in brain and skin.[9]

Cystolic retinoic acid-binding proteins (CRABPs)

This protein, found in the cytosol, has a molecular mass of around 15 kDa. The inter-species conservation of the amino acid sequence is high, particularly in the amino acid terminal region. CRABP also shows extensive homology with other proteins which bind and transport hydrophobic substances, the most notable being the CRBPs described above, a peripheral nerve myelin protein 2, fatty acid-binding protein (FABP) and liver protein Z.[10]

Distribution of CRABP is ubiquitous and relatively large amounts have been detected in testes, uterus, eye and epidermis. It is also expressed in many cell lines, but a notable exception is the human myeloleukaemia line HL60. Expression of CRABP is controlled by RA.[11] Recently, two different isoforms of CRABP (I and II) have been found in neonatal rats. CRABP II was present in significant amounts only in the skin and most of the CRABP I was found in the same tissue. As shown in Table 2.1, RA has different affinities for CRABP I and CRABP II ($K_d = 4.2 \times 10^{-9}$M (rat testis)[13] and 6.5×10^{-8}M (neonatal rat skin),[12] respectively).

Nuclear retinoic acid receptors

From the cytosol, the retinoid is delivered to its presumed site of action, the nucleus. Several specific RA receptor proteins (RARs) have been identified.[14–18] The structural organization of these RARs is similar to that of the steroid and thyroid hormone receptor family and, in common with the other members of this superfamily, the RARs are composed of three distinct domains: ligand binding, DNA binding and gene transactivation. The three RAR proteins show a high degree of homology in amino acid sequence not only in the DNA but also in the ligand-binding domain. However, there are wide differences in amino acid sequence in amino- and carboxy-terminal regions. It was through these proteins belonging to the superfamily of hormone transactivating factors, which possess high homology in the cysteine-rich DNA-binding domain, that the RAR family was originally identified using the 'finger swapping' technique.[14] The molecular mass of these receptors is about 50 kDa and the human proteins known as hRAR-α, hRAR-β and hRAR-γ contain 462, 445 and 454 amino acids, respectively (Figure 2.2).

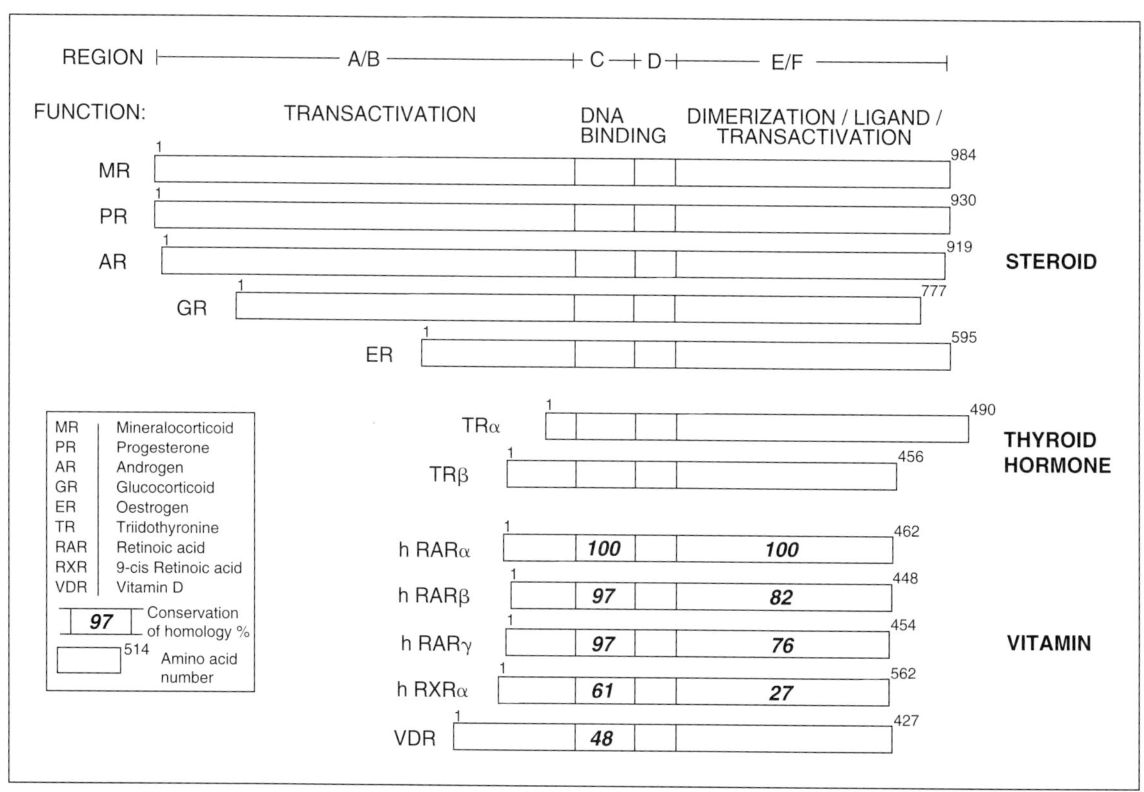

Figure 2.2

Nuclear receptor gene superfamily.

In contrast, a nuclear receptor (RXR) that identifies a novel RA response pathway has been described in which the homology with RARs in both the DNA and ligand-binding domains is low.[19] The naturally occurring 9-*cis*-RA binds and activates the RXRs and RARs. The all-*trans* isomer of RA (AtRA) binds and activates the RARs only.[20–24] X-ray crystallographic analysis and molecular modelling studies suggest that, when retinoic acid binds to its receptor, the latter undergoes conformational changes preventing the ligand from dissociating readily.[21]

Following ligand binding, the accessory proteins may be co-activators[22] or co-repressors.[23] These factors are believed to be released (co-repressor) or bound (co-activator) following the conformational change elicited by the ligand on the receptor. The above mechanisms are termed direct as they involve ligand–RAR/RXR–DNA interaction. Retinoid ligands can also act indirectly by antagonizing the interaction of other transcription factors with DNA. AP-1 is a protein complex (c-Jun/c-Fos) regulating cell proliferation. By forming 'false dimers', such as c-Jun-RAR which is unable to bind to DNA response elements specific for retinoid or AP-1, a retinoid may antagonize the proliferative response that follows induction of AP-1.[24]

The discovery of several isoforms of each RAR generated by alternative RNA splicing has complicated the understanding of this complex field in that these proteins are differentially expressed both spatially and temporally, that is, in terms of the tissue and stage of morphological development of the species.[25,26]

Action of retinoids on the target cell

Within the context of this chapter, in order to appreciate the mode of action of retinoids a number of limitations will be defined. First, only naturally occurring retinoids will be included as the transport and binding interaction of the numerous synthetic derivatives is poorly defined. Thus, retinol, RA, vitamin A_2 acid and their metabolites will be considered. Second, very few human data are available and many of the intracellular binding data relate to neonatal mouse, chick embryo and a plethora of cells in culture. Great care must be exercised when extrapolating from one study to another. The striking, sometimes paradoxical effects of retinoids on cell differentiation and pattern formation in embryogenesis would suggest that their molecular action is itself quite complex. In essence, since the retinoids, the binding proteins and the gene targets are conserved within the species, the biological control mechanism involved in the retinoid area may also operate with other members of the superfamily (Figure 2.2). It is likely that we are dealing with a biological control mechanism of more general applicability.

CRBP I and CRBP II can carry retinol in vivo to intracellular sites of action and metabolism. The enzyme currently believed to be responsible for retinol esterification is located in the microsomal fraction of liver and intestine and is termed lecithin retinol acyl transferase (LRAT).[27] The retinol–CRBP I and retinol–CRBP II complexes (holoform) are effective substrates for LRAT but, in contrast, these holoproteins are not esterified by acyl-CoA retinol transferase (ARAT). No nuclear interactions with retinol or RBPs have yet been described. Thus, at present it is assumed that the physiological role of retinol or its esters is that of a regulated source of retinoic acid (except in vision).

There exists an effective mechanism for the re-conversion of retinyl esters to retinol.[28] Retinol ester hydrolase (REH) activity is mainly present in the liver but has also been detected in several other tissues. Two types of hydrolase exist. The most widely studied is a neutral REH activity which can be stimulated by millimolar concentrations of bile salts. The activity is located in the nuclear fraction of rat liver homogenates. Another REH activity has been reported in the membrane fraction and functions independently of bile salts. There is considerable evidence to support the idea that retinol is effectively transformed into RA by different tissue homogenates or cells in culture.[29] It is noteworthy that this activity is maintained in the presence of inhibitors of ethanol metabolism. The oxidation occurs in fractions of differentiating keratinocytes in culture or psoriatic plaques, but not in normal human skin or non-differentiated keratinocytes in culture.[30] The levels of a new metabolite of retinol [4-hydroxy-4,14-retro-retinol (4 HRR)] were elevated in human skin following topical application of retinol under occlusion. In contrast to vitamin A, 4-HRR did not produce characteristic cutaneous retinoid responses.[31]

In essence, the cell itself possesses effective tools to modulate the major precursor of RA. The importance of this for the spatial–temporal effects of retinoid action is developed below.

To summarize the above, the role of the plasma-binding proteins is to deliver retinol in a free or esterified form to its cellular target. At the cellular level the holoproteins can deliver their ligand for further biotransformation, either to be stored in an esterified form, or to be oxidized to RA. In addition, the cell can hydrolyse the ester back to retinol. This process supplies a major control element in retinoid physiology, because these binding proteins are differentially expressed in tissues during differentiation and embryogenesis. Although metabolism is not the theme of this chapter, the report that RA production from retinol (via retinaldehyde) can be inhibited by RA[29] supports the idea that retinoid gradients can be created in different tissues at different times. This is supported by the recent evidence that expression of alcohol dehydrogenase enzyme type III is modulated by interaction of RA with RA response elements (RARE).[32] RAREs show diad symmetries and are usually found in the promoter region of retinoid-responsive genes. This idea gained ground following the elegant and detailed studies of Thallar and Eichele,[33] who proposed that RA is a morphogen and is responsible for specifying positional information during embryogenesis. They measured the RA concentration in chick developing limb bud and found that there exists a concentration gradient with the highest concentration in the posterior region. If exogenous RA is applied to the anterior region, a mirror of the biological effect (digit duplication) observed at the posterior region is observed. Thallar and Eichele report that the RA concentration ranges from about 20 nM at the anterior site to 50 nM at the posterior site. In view of the potency of RA (1–10 nM) the tissue and cell must be able to exercise gradient control and bioavailability very precisely.

How can the bioavailability of the proposed morphogen be more finely controlled? An attractive hypothesis involves CRABP. From in situ hybridization,[34,35] immunohistochemical[36,37] and direct binding studies[36] in mouse and chick embryos, expression of CRABP was localized to tissues derived from the neural crest. These are the tissues that are particularly affected in RA embryopathy. In the limb bud, high levels of CRABP were observed at sites where local RA levels are low and, conversely, low levels of CRABP were detected at the posterior limb bud margin where the morphogen concentration is low.[34,38] Thus, a concentration gradient of CRABP within a given tissue would serve to amplify the gradient of RA by controlling the free amount available for interaction with the nuclear receptors. Recent data, however, do not fully confirm the gradient theory. It is proposed that RA may induce phenotypic modifications in a mesenchymal cell group, which in turn, by as yet undefined mediators, relays the biological signals to the adjacent developing tissue.[39,40]

As indicated earlier, this is a simplified picture of a most complex process. The roles of halo- and apo-CRABP I and II, CRBP I and CRBP II are not fully understood. Their respective expression patterns need to be studied in more detail, and since the dissociation constants for their respective ligands, RA and retinol, differ by at least one order of magnitude, knowledge of the active concentration present at a given 'bioavailability' site is lacking.

The next stage in the action of retinoids, or more precisely their carboxylic acid derivatives, is the interaction with the nuclear RA receptors (RARs, RXRs). An unanswered fundamental question is why would nature control cell differentiation by imposing at least three types of proteins, each with several isoforms, which specifically recognize one ligand? Part of the answer is revealed by the results of recent studies that show that the receptors themselves, which are transcription factors, can regulate the expression not only of structural proteins but also of other transcription factors. The fact that all three RAR proteins are not co-expressed in all tissues suggests that the ability of a cell to express one or several of these proteins controls the sensitivity and nature of the response of a given cell or tissue to RA. However, to date only a few RAREs have been identified. Growth hormone, laminin and alcohol dehydrogenase type III, in addition to RAR-β, are unregulated by RA–RAR complexes.[32,41–44] The difficulty is further compounded by the notion that RA–RAR complexes may also suppress the expression of other transcription factors. The presence of the RA is not mandatory to form the RAR–DNA in vitro complex; however, the ligand is deemed necessary for gene activation.[38] The natural ligand may not be essential at this late stage in the cascade of events, but in view of the limited number of RAREs identified this explanation should be accepted cautiously. RXRs play a key role in that they can mediate via heterodimers the activity of a number of hormone receptors that are activated by structurally unrelated ligands. The receptor–DNA complex determines the retinoid response.[45]

Another important question focuses on retinol: is it simply a prohormone or are there as yet unidentified receptors for this ligand? Finally, retinoid analogues exist which have different binding characteristics to those of the natural ligands.[46,47] Further studies with these ligands and correlating their binding selectivities and affinities with gene control, pharmacological and toxicological properties will help increase our knowledge in this area, in which spectacular progress has already been made in the recent past.

The relevance of this work to clinical practice is two-fold. First, the use of retinoids in the treatment of skin disease is extensive[48] and a better understanding of their transport, distribution and mode of action will lead to the design of better and safer therapies. Second, it has recently been reported that genomic rearrangement occurs in cell lines derived from patients suffering from acute promyelocytic leukaemia (APL). The RAR-α gene has been translocated from chromosome 17 to a locus *myl*/RAR-α fusion mRNA.[49] Thus abnormal expression of genes coding for transactivating factors such as RARs may well be linked to the aetiology of certain malignant diseases.

A quantitative analysis of the distribution of retinoids in different skin layers in samples from healthy subjects revealed that a concentration gradient of retinol and dehydroretinol (vitamin A_2) exists, the major proportion occurring in the epidermis as opposed to the dermis. The role of vitamin A_2 (dehydroretinol) and its metabolites warrants further study as this substance is found in relatively high proportions in normal skin.[5] In addition, variations in vitamin A and vitamin A_2 levels have been reported in a variety of skin disorders.[50,51] The affinity of the vitamin A_2 series for the key intra- and extracellular receptors needs to be determined.

There is a need to examine further retinoid gradients within the epidermis. In a model system it has been shown that RA markedly affects the morphogenesis of epidermis reconstructed on a collagen matrix seeded with human fibroblasts.[52] At 10^{-8} M RA concentration a fully differentiated (orthokeratotic) epidermis was obtained. In the absence of RA or at the higher concentration of 10^{-7} M, hyperkeratotic or parakeratotic tissue was obtained, respectively.

A role for these binding proteins in psoriasis has been suggested. In normal skin, CRAPB I and II are expressed in a ratio of 1:1.4, and there exists some evidence to suggest that there is a marked over-expression of CRAPB II in psoriatic lesions.[60–63] The genes encoding RAR-α, -β, -γ are present in human skin. In the epidermis in particular, RAR-γ predominates with only low levels of RAR-α. In the dermal fibroblast all three subtypes are expressed and in addition RAR-β is also induced by AtRA. RXR-α is the most highly expressed receptor type in the skin and the RAR-γ/RXR-α heterodimer has been shown to be potentially the active transcription regulator in human skin.[61] The importance of retinoic acid receptors in skin structure and function was demonstrated by targeting the expression of a dominant negative retinoic acid receptor mutant in the epidermis of transgenic mice.[62] These RAR-α 'impaired' mice exhibited a marked phenotype of red shiny skin. Compared with normal control animals a faster rate of transepidermal water loss and a thinner more loosely packed stratum corneum were observed. Electron microscopic examination revealed abnormalities in intracellular lipids.

Finally, an example of the indirect retinoid receptor mechanism was demonstrated in the skin.[63] It was shown that AtRA applied prior to irradiation with low doses of UVB substantially reduced the induction of AP-1 and related metalloproteinases . This provides a molecular model for aspects of skin photodamage in that the expression and function of metalloproteinases which degrade extracellular matrix proteins such as collagen and elastin are modulated by AP-1.

In this chapter, the complex process of transport, distribution and action of retinoids has been reviewed. This area is rapidly evolving and so the view of some details such as those of nuclear interactions will certainly alter in the future. The relevance, however, of the key features highlighted here to retinoid physiology and pharmacology is evident.

Acknowledgment

The author would like to thank Bernard Martin for his help in the preparation of the table and figures.

References

1. McCollum EV, Davis M, The nature of the dietary deficiencies of rice. *J Biol Chem* (1915) **23**: 181–91.
2. Wald G, Carotenoids and the visual cycle. *J Gen Physiol* (1935) **19**: 351–61.
3. Hennekens CH, Mayrent SL, Willet W, Vitamin A, carotenoids and retinoids. *Cancer* (1986) **58**: 1837–41.
4. Napoli JL, Race KR, Biogenesis of retinoic acid from β-carotene. *J Biol Chem* (1988) **263**: 17372–7.
5. Vahlquist A, Lee JB, Michaëlsson G et al, Vitamin A in human skin: II concentrations of carotene, retinol and dehydroretinol in various components of normal skin. *J Invest Dermatol* (1982) **79**: 94–7.
6. Blaner WS, Goodman WS de, Purification and properties of plasma retinol binding protein. *Methods Enzymol* (1991) **190**: 193–206.
7. Ong DE, Vitamin A-binding proteins. *Nutr Rev* (1985) **43**: 225–32.
8. Levin MS, Li E, Ong DE et al, Comparison of the tissue-specific expression and development regulation of two closely linked rodent

genes encoding cystolic retinol-binding proteins. *J Biol Chem* (1987) **262**: 7118–24.
9. Kato M, Blaner WS, Mertz JR et al, Influence of retinoid nutritional status of cellular retinol- and cellular retinoic acid-binding protein concentrations in various rat tissues. *J Biol Chem* (1985) **260**: 4832–8.
10. Sundelin J, Das SR, Erikson U et al, The primary structure of bovine cellular retinoic acid-binding protein. *J Biol Chem* (1985) **260**: 6494–9.
11. Siegenthaler G, Saurat JH, Plasma and skin carriers for natural and synthetic retinoids. *Arch Dermatol* (1987) **123**: 1690 (abstract).
12. Bailey JS, Siu C-H, Purification and partial characterization of a novel binding protein for retinoic acid from neonatal rat. *J Biol Chem* (1988) **263**: 9326–32.
13. Ong DE, Chytil F, Cellular retinoic acid-binding protein from rat testis. Purification and characterization. *J Biol Chem* (1978) **253**: 4551–4.
14. Petkovich M, Brand NJ, Krust A et al, A human retinoic acid receptor which belongs to the family of nuclear receptors. *Nature* (1987) **330**: 444–50.
15. Giguere V, Ong ES, Segui P et al, Identification of a receptor for the morphogen retinoic acid. *Nature* (1988) **330**: 624–9.
16. Brand N, Petkovich M, Krust A et al, Identification of a second retinoic acid receptor. *Nature* (1988) **332**: 850–3.
17. Benbrook D, Lernhardt E, Pfahl M, A new retinoic acid receptor identified from a hepato-cellular carcinoma. *Nature* (1988) **333**: 669–72.
18. Krust A, Kastner P, Petkovich M et al, A third human retinoic acid receptor hRARgamma. *Proc Natl Acad Sci USA* (1989) **86**: 5310–14.
19. Mangelsdorf DJ, Ong ES, Dyck JA et al, Nuclear receptor that identifies a novel retinoic acid response pathway. *Nature* (1990) **345**: 224–9.
20. Levin AA, Strurzenbecker LJ, Kazmer S et al, 9-cis-Retinoic acid stereoisomer binds and activates the nuclear receptor RXR-α. *Nature* (1992) **355**: 359–66.
21. Wurtz JM, Bourget W, Renaud JP et al, A canonical structure for the ligand binding domain of Nuclear Receptors. *Nat Struct Biol* (1996) **3**: 87–94.
22. Cavailles V, Dauvois S, L'Horset F et al, Nuclear Factor RIP 40 modulates transcriptional activation by the estrogen receptor. *EMBO J* (1995) **14**: 3741–51.
23. Chen D, Evans R, A Transcriptional co-repressor that interacts with nuclear hormone receptors. *Nature* (1995) **377**:454–7.
24. Pfahl M, Nuclear receptor/AP-1 Interaction. *Endocrinol Rev* (1993) **14**: 651–8.
25. Leroy P, Krust A, Zelent A et al, Multiple isoforms of the mouse retinoic acid receptor α are generated by alternative splicing and differential induction by retinoic acid. *EMBO J* (1991) **10**: 59–69.
26. Zelent A, Mendelsohn C, Kastner P et al, Differentially expressed isoforms of the mouse retinoic acid receptor β are generated by usage of two promoters and alternative splicing. *EMBO J* (1991) **10**: 71–81.
27. MacDonald PN, Ong DE, Assay of lecithin–retinol acyltransferase. *Methods Enzymol* (1990) **189**: 450–9.
28. Harrison EH, Napoli JL, Bile salt-independent retinyl ester hydrolase activities associated with membranes of rat tissues. *Methods Enzymol* (1990) **189**: 459–69.
29. Siegenthaler G, Saurant J-H, Ponec M, The formation of retinoic acid from retinol in relation to the differentiation state of cultured human keratinocytes. *Pharmacol Skin* (1989) **3**: 52–5.
30. Siegenthaler G, Gumowski-Sunek D, Saurat J-H, Metabolism of natural retinoids in psoriatic epidermis. *J Invest Dermatol* (1990) **95**: 47S–48S.
31. Duell E A, Derguini F, Sewan K et al, Extraction of human epidermis treated with retinol yields *retro* retinoids in addition to free retinol and retinyl esters. *J Invest Dermatol* (1996) **107**: 178–82
32. Duester G, Shean ML, McBride M et al, Retinoic acid response element in the human alcohol dehydrogenase gene ADH3: implications for regulation of retinoic acid synthesis. *Mol Cell Biol* (1991) **11**: 1638–46.
33. Thaller C, Eichele G, Identification and spatial distribution of retinoids in the developing chick limb bud. *Nature* (1987) **327**: 625–8.
34. Perez-Castro AV, Toth-Rogler LE, Wie L-N et al, Spatial and temporal pattern of expression of the cellular retinoic acid-binding protein

and the cellular retinol-binding protein during mouse embryogenesis. *Proc Natl Acad Sci USA* (1989) **86**: 8813–17.

35. Vaessen M-J, Miejers JHC, Bootsma D et al, The cellular retinoic acid-binding protein is expressed in tissues associated with retinoic-acid-induced malformation. *Development* (1990) **110**: 371–8.
36. Dencker L, Annarwall E, Busch C et al, Localization of specific retinoid-binding sites and expression of cellular retinoic-acid-binding protein (CRABP) in the early mouse embryo. *Development* (1990) **110**: 343–52.
37. Maden M, Ong DE, Chytil F, Retinoid-binding protein distribution in the developing mammalian nervous system. *Development* (1990) **109**: 75–80.
38. Maden M, Ong DE, Summerbell D et al, Spatial distribution of cellular protein binding to retinoic acid in the chick limb bud. *Nature* (1988) **335**: 733–5.
39. Wanek N, Gardiner DM, Muneoka K et al, Conversion by retinoic acid of anterior cells into ZPA cells in the chick wing bud. *Nature* (1991) **350**: 81–3.
40. Noji S, Nohno T, Koama E et al, Retinoic acid induces polarizing activity but is likely to be a morphogen in the chick limb bud. *Nature* (1991) **350**: 83–6.
41. Bedo G, Stantisteban P, Aranda A, Retinoic acid regulates growth hormone gene expression. *Nature* (1989) **339**: 231–4.
42. Vasios GW, Gold JD, Petkovich M et al, A retinoic acid-responsive element is present in the 5′-flanking region of the laminin B_1 gene. *Proc Natl Acad Sci USA* (1989) **86**: 9099–103.
43. De Thé H, Vivanco-Ruiz MDM, Tiollais P et al, Identification of a retinoic acid responsive element in the retinoic acid receptor beta gene. *Nature* (1990) **343**: 177–80.
44. Astrom A Petterson U, Chambon P, Retinoic acid induction of human cellular retinoic acid binding protein II gene transcription is mediated by retinoic acid receptor--retinoid X receptor heterodimers bound to one far upstream retinoic acid-responsive element with 5 base pair spacing. *J Biol Chem* (1994) **269**: 22334–9.
45. La Vista-Picard N, Hobbs PD, Pfahl M, The receptor DNA complex determines the retinoid response: a mechanism for the diversification of the ligand signal. *Mol Cell Biol* (1996) **16**: 4137–46.
46. Darmon M, Rocher M, Cavey M-T et al, Biological activity of retinoids correlates with affinity for nuclear receptors, but not for cytosolic binding protein. *Skin Pharmacol* (1988) **1**: 161–75.
47. Shroot B, A strategy for discovery of new retinoid-like substances. *Pharmacol Skin* (1989) **3**: 270–7.
48. Saurat J-H, Clinical pharmacology of systemic retinoids. *Pharmacol Skin* (1989) **3**: 215–26.
49. De Thé H, Chomienne C, Lanotte M et al, The T(15;17) translocation of acute promyelocytic leukaemia fuses the retinoic acid receptor a gene to a novel transcribed locus. *Nature* (1990) **347**: 558–60.
50. Rollman O, Vahlquist A, Cutaneous vitamin A levels in seborrhoeic keratosis, actinic keratosis and basal cell carcinoma. *Arch Dermatol Res* (1981) **270**: 193–6.
51. Vahlquist A, Törmä H, Rollman O et al, Distribution of natural and synthetic retinoids in the skin. In: Saurant J-H. (ed). *Retinoids: new trends in research and therapy*. Karger: Basel, 1985, 159–67.
52. Asselineau D, Bernard BA, Bailly C et al, Retinoic acid improves the morphogenesis of human epidermis in vitro. *Dev Biol* (1989) **133**: 322–35.
53. Bonelli FC, de Luca LMA, a high performance liquid chromatographic technique that separates cellular retinol binding protein from cellular retinoic acid binding protein. *Anal Biochem* (1985) **147**: 251–7.
54. Ong DE, Chytil F, Cellular retinol-binding protein from rat liver. *J Biol Chem* (1987) **253**: 828–32.
55. Noy N, Zu ZJ, Interactions of retinol with binding proteins: implications for the mechanism of uptake by cells. *Biochemistry* (1990) **29**: 3878–83.
56. Chertow BS, Moore MR, Blaner W et al, Cytoplasmic retinoid-binding proteins and retinoid effects on insulin release in $RINm_5F$ β-cells. *Diabetes* (1989) **38**: 1544–8.
57. Crettaz M, Baron A, Siegenthaler G et al, Ligand specificities of recombinant retinoic acid receptors RARα and RARβ. *Biochem J* (1990) **272**: 391–7.

58. Howard WB, Sharma RP, Willhite CC et al, Binding affinities of retinoids to fetal cellular retinoic acid binding protein (CRABP) in relation to their teratogenic potency in hamsters. *Biochem Pharmacol* (1990) **40**: 643–8.
59. Jetten AM, Grippo JF, Nervi C, Isolation and binding characteristics of nuclear retinoic acid receptors. *Methods Enzymol* (1991) **189**: 248–55.
60. Siegenthaler G, Tomatis I, Chatellard-Gruaz D et al, Expression of CRAPB I and II in human epidermal cells. Alteration of relative protein amounts is linked to the state of differentiation. *Biochem J* (1992) **287**: 383–9.
61. Fisher GJ, Harvinder ST, Jia-Hao X et al, Immunological identification and functional quantitation of retinoic acid and retinoic X receptor proteins in human skin. *J Biol Chem* (1994) **269**: 20629–35.
62. Imakado S, Bickenbach JR, Bundman DS et al, Targeting expression of a dominant negative retinoic acid receptor mutant in the epidermis of transgenic mice results in loss of barrier function. *Genes and Development* (1995) **9**: 317–29.
63. Fisher GJ, Datta SC, Talwar HS et al, Molecular basis for sun-induced premature skin aging and retinoid antagonism. *Nature* (1996) **379**: 335–9.

3 Retinoid nuclear receptors

Roshantha AS Chandraratna and Elliott S Klein

Introduction

Retinoids are small, fat-soluble molecules that include vitamin A_1 (retinol) and numerous natural and synthetic derivatives. The requirement of retinoids for normal cellular growth, differentiation, vision, reproduction and other vital functions in the adult have been recognized since the classical studies on vitamin A deficiency by Wolbach and Howe.[1,2] The molecular basis of vitamin A action in vision was originally elucidated by Wald[3] and co-workers, and details regarding the interaction of 11-*cis*-retinal, the visual chromophore, with opsin, the visual pigment protein, and the processes of visual transduction and adaptation are now well understood.[4] However, the molecular mechanisms by which retinoids elicit their numerous other biological effects remained unelucidated until the recent breakthrough discovery of nuclear retinoid receptors.[5,6] These nuclear receptors are ligand-activated transcription factors that regulate the expression of genes. It is now generally accepted that the vast majority of the non-visual functions of retinoids are effected by gene regulatory mechanisms via their cognate nuclear receptors. Thus, although the classification of physiological retinoids as vitamins still holds because of their dietary origin, retinoids can also be termed hormones similar to the steroid and thyroid hormones. In this chapter, we broadly review the current state of knowledge of retinoid nuclear receptors and the mechanisms of hormone activation and gene regulation.

Retinoid receptors

There are six known retinoid receptors, which belong to two distinct families: the retinoic acid receptors (RARs) and the retinoid X receptors (RXRs).[7] The nomenclature for the receptors is derived from the activating hormones associated with them. Thus the physiological hormone for the RARs is *trans*-retinoic acid (RA), which is an oxidative metabolite of vitamin A_1.[5] At the time of the discovery of the first RXR,[8] the activating hormone (retinoid X) was not known, although it was believed to be a derivative of RA. It has been subsequently shown that 9-*cis*-retinoic acid (9-*cis*-RA), a geometric isomer and derivative of RA, is a high-affinity activator of RXRs.[9,10] However, the evidence for 9-*cis*-RA being a physiological hormone for RXRs remains unconvincing. The RAR and RXR families each consist of three subtypes (α, β and γ), themselves the products of distinct genes.[7] There are also

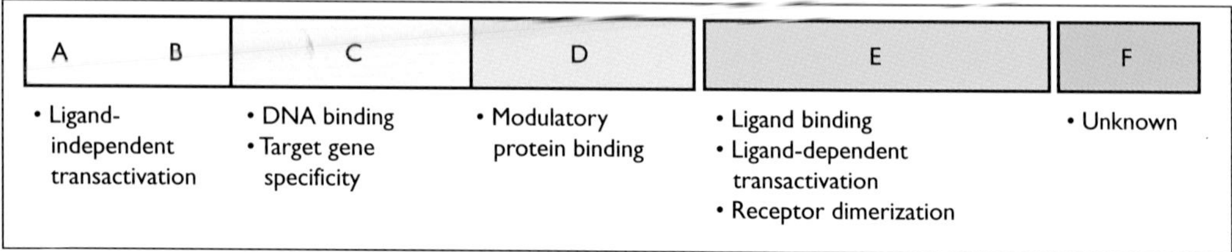

Figure 3.1

Modular structure and functions of RAR proteins.

multiple isoforms for these subtypes that are generated by alternative splicing and by differential use of promoters. These subtypes and isoforms are variably expressed in humans in a tissue- and cell-specific manner. For example, the major RAR and RXR subtypes present in adult human skin are RAR-γ and RXR-α.[11]

The retinoid receptors belong to a superfamily of nuclear receptors that include the steroid, vitamin D and thyroid receptors, among others. All of these receptors have evolved from a primordial gene, and accordingly have very similar structures that are conserved across species. Nuclear receptors are modular in their structure, with each module having different functions. Similar modules can actually be interchanged between receptors by genetic engineering techniques, with retention of function of the modules in the resulting chimaeric protein. For example, the RAR proteins consist of six functionally different modules, which are labelled regions A–F (Figure 3.1).[12] The A/B region has a gene transactivation function that does not require binding of hormone for activity. The C region encodes a cysteine-rich DNA-binding domain (DBD). Coordinate binding of these cysteine residues with zinc generates the so-called 'zinc fingers', which make contact with DNA. 'Zinc finger' is actually a misnomer, since X-ray crystallographic analysis indicates that the cysteine–zinc coordinate binding actually provides the neccessary tertiary arrangement of α-helical domains within the DBD to make specific contact with DNA. The D region has recently been shown to interact with other nuclear proteins that modulate RAR activity. The E region contains the ligand-binding domain (LBD), a hormone-dependent transactivation function and a hydrophobic zipper region that is responsible for receptor dimerization. The F region, for which the function is unknown, is absent in RXR proteins. Alignment of the amino acid sequences of the members of the nuclear receptor superfamily indicates a variable degree of conservation within these domains. The C region, which contains the DBD, is the most highly conserved, while the E region, which contains the LBDs, is quite divergent. The variability in the LBDs has an important physiological significance, since it enables the different receptors to be specifically recognized and activated by only their corresponding hormones.

Mechanisms of retinoid receptor action

The nuclear retinoid receptors are ligand-dependent transcription factors that regulate the expression of a wide range of target genes. The retinoid receptors are located primarily in the nuclei of cells and in many instances require hormone binding for activation.

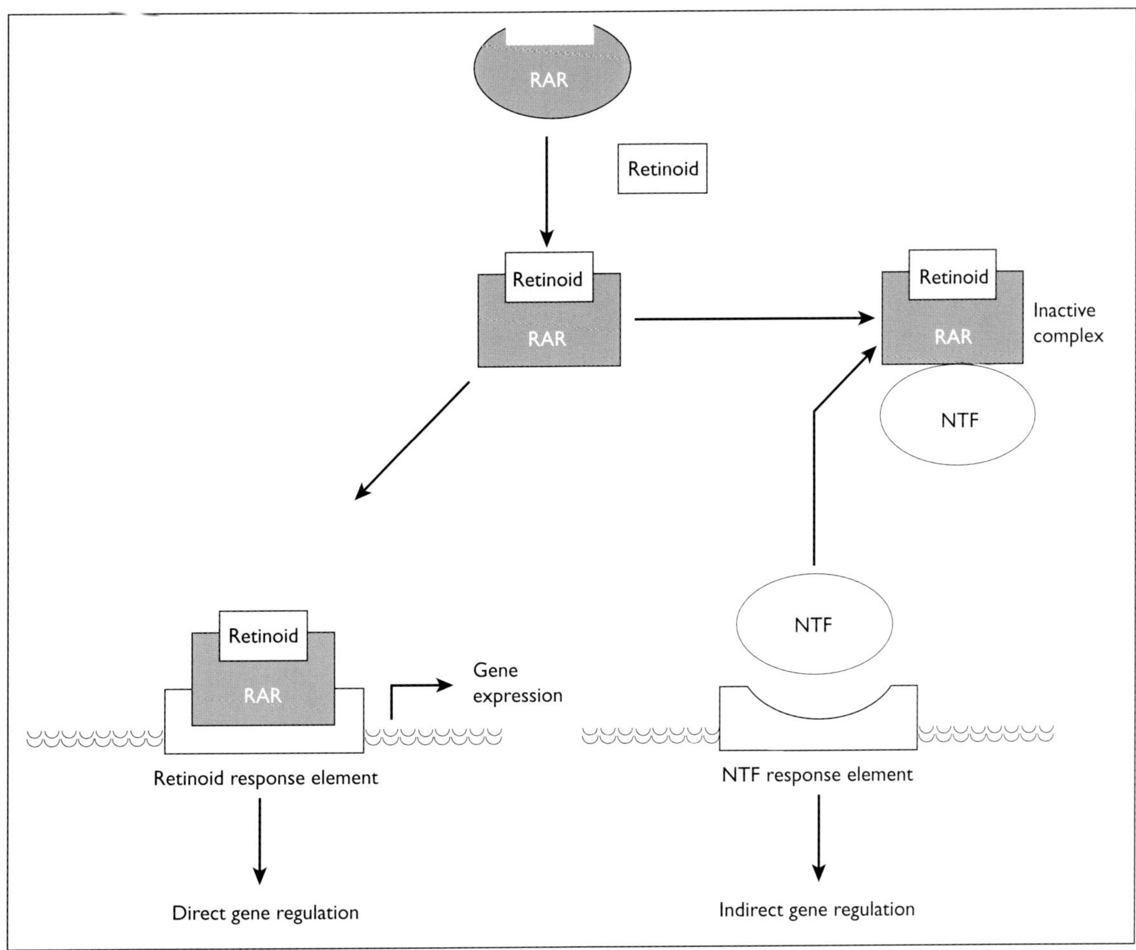

Figure 3.2

General mechanisms of retinoid receptor gene regulation.

Binding of hormone to the receptor causes a conformational change of the receptor to its 'activated' form. The hormone-bound receptor can interact with a different set of nuclear proteins, including intermediary proteins and members of the transcriptional complex, than the unoccupied receptor. The activated retinoid–receptor complexes can regulate gene transcription in two distinct ways:

(a) they can bind directly to retinoid receptor response elements in the promoter regions of target genes and regulate the transcription of these genes; or
(b) they can antagonize the action of other nuclear transcription factors (NTFs), such as AP-1, and regulate the expression of genes that are controlled by these transcription factors (Figure 3.2).

The latter mechanism can involve direct interaction of retinoid receptor with an NTF, leading to an inactive complex as shown in Figure 3.2. Alternatively, the retinoid receptor can sequester an intermediary protein that is required for the function of the NTF and thereby antagonize its function. It is possible to up-regulate or down-regulate the expression of genes by either mechanism.

Receptor dimerization: RXR as master regulator

Although the simplified cartoon in Figure 3.2 shows a single RAR binding to a response element, high-affinity binding of these nuclear receptors to DNA is obtained only as dimers. In vivo, RARs always bind to their cognate response elements as RAR–RXR heterodimers.[13] With three subtypes in each family, there are nine possible permutations of RAR–RXR heterodimers, and while this raises the possibility that each of these combinations may have distinct physiological roles, some level of functional redundancy appears to be the case. The RXRs can also form transcriptionally active RXR–RXR homodimers in the presence of RXR ligands,[14] but the in vivo relevance of these homodimers has not been clearly established. The steroid hormone receptors, on the other hand, always function as homodimers. The vitamin D receptor (VDR), thyroid receptor (TR), peroxisome proliferator-activated receptor (PPAR) and some 'orphan' receptors also form heterodimers with RXRs. Thus RXRs are required for the direct gene regulatory activities of RARs, VDR, TR and PPAR, and appear to act as master regulators of all of these hormonal pathways. Interestingly, activation of these heterodimeric hormonal pathways requires ligand binding only to the non-RXR component of the heterodimer, with the RXR acting as a 'silent partner'. It is very clear that binding of a ligand only to the RAR portion of an RAR–RXR heterodimer fully activates RAR hormonal pathways in vivo. However, there is recent evidence to suggest that binding of RXR ligands to the RXR portion of the heterodimer can modulate RAR ligand activity.[15] Similarly, the activation of VDR, TR and PPAR hormonal pathways by specific ligands can also be potentially affected by RXR ligands.[16]

Response element specificity: how nuclear receptors target different genes

An important question in physiology is: how do members of the nuclear receptor superfamily achieve target gene selectivity? That is, why do RARs, VDR and glucocorticoid receptors, for example, regulate quite distinct sets of genes? These dimeric nuclear receptors actually recognize pairs of consensus sequences of nucleotides of six bases, referred to as 'half-sites'. The consensus nucleotide sequence for the steroid receptors is AGAACA, while that for the retinoid/thyroid receptor subfamily is AGGTCA. The specificity of this protein–DNA interaction is quite high, and provides the first level of differentiation in the way that different nuclear receptors can find their target genes. Only five amino acids within the DBD, designated the proximal box (P-box), confer this specificity in half-site recognition. In fact, the mutation of the P-box of either the RAR or RXR to that of the glucocorticoid receptor results in a retinoid receptor that now recognizes a glucocorticoid response element half-site.[17] A second level of differentiation is introduced in the manner in which the consensus sequences are arranged in the promoter regions of various genes. In the case

Dimer pair	Response element	Consensus sequence
RXR RXR →1→	DR-1	AGGTCA
RXR PPAR →1→	DR-1	AGGTCA
RXR RAR →2→	DR-2	AGGTCA
RXR VDR →3→	DR-3	AGGTCA
RXR TR →4→	DR-4	AGGTCA
RXR RAR →5→	DR-5	AGGTCA
GR GR →3←	palindrome	AGAACA

Figure 3.3

Response element specificity for nuclear receptor dimers.

of the homodimeric steroid receptors, the consensus sequences are arranged as palindromes to form steroid response elements. For the heterodimeric receptor pairs, such as RAR–RXR, the consensus sequences are arranged as direct repeats (DR). Thus the symmetrically paired steroid receptors, which dimerize in a head-to-head manner, can readily recognize and bind to the symmetrically arranged palindromic response elements. On the other hand, the asymmetrical heterodimeric receptor pairs (e.g. RAR–RXR), which dimerize in a head-to-tail manner, can bind with high affinity only to the asymmetrical direct repeat response elements.

The next question is: how do the various heterodimeric receptors, such as RAR–RXR and VDR–RXR, differentiate between their target genes? The answer appears to lie in the 'spacer rule', which states that the heterodimer response element specificity is derived largely from the number of nucleotides that separate the two consensus sequences in a direct repeat response element.[18] Thus RAR–RXR heterodimers specifically bind to and activate direct repeat response elements that are separated by 2 (DR-2) or 5 (DR-5) nucleotides (Figure 3.3). Retinoid-responsive genes, which are regulated by direct binding of retinoid receptors, contain, for the most part, DR-2 or DR-5 response elements in their promoter regions. The corresponding RXR heterodimers for PPAR, VDR and TR selectively recognize DR-1, DR-3 and DR-4 response elements respectively. The RXR–RXR homodimers constitute an apparent exception to the above rules, since in transfected cells they can bind to and activate transcription from DR-1 response elements. However, the physiological relevance of RXR homodimer activation of DR-1 elements is unclear, since recent studies suggest that RXR homodimers do not exist in vivo even in tissues where there are high levels of RXR protein.[11] These phenomena of specific response element recognition by different nuclear receptor dimers account for the ability of the various nuclear receptor hormonal pathways to target distinct sets of genes and produce unique physiological responses.

Co-activators and co-repressors and how RARs get turned on

It is clear that the binding of hormone to a nuclear receptor must cause some change in the shape of the receptor, resulting in it being 'activated'. What type of conformational change occurs upon ligand binding? How does this shape change lead to receptor 'activation'? These are the type of fundamental questions that are being addressed in current research on nuclear receptors. A recent set of papers has gone a long way to answering the first question regarding the type of conformational change that occurs upon hormone binding. The crystal structure of unliganded RXR-α LBD reveals a structure containing 12 α-helices, which are arranged in three layers.[19] One of the helices, helix 12, protrudes away from the rest of the receptor and exposes a hydrophobic cavity, which is believed to be the ligand-binding pocket. The crystal structures of RAR-γ[20] and TR[21] with the corresponding hormones, RA and thyroid hormone, bound within them have also been recently determined. Comparison of the unliganded RXR-α and the liganded RAR-γ and TR LBDs have yielded a wealth of information regarding conformational changes in the receptor upon ligand binding. Overall, ligand binding induces a more compact, stable structure in the receptor. The most striking specific change that occurs is that helix 12 folds over and covers the entry to the hydrophobic ligand-binding pocket, thereby 'trapping' the ligand within the pocket. The binding of RA to RAR-γ has been likened to the action of a mousetrap, whereby RA (the mouse) is drawn into the ligand-binding pocket (the trap) by the electrostatic potential of the receptor, and the resultant conformational change involving movement of helix 12 to close the pocket constitutes the springing of the trap. This mechanism then generates the next question as to how the ligand gets out. While a permanently trapped mouse may be a

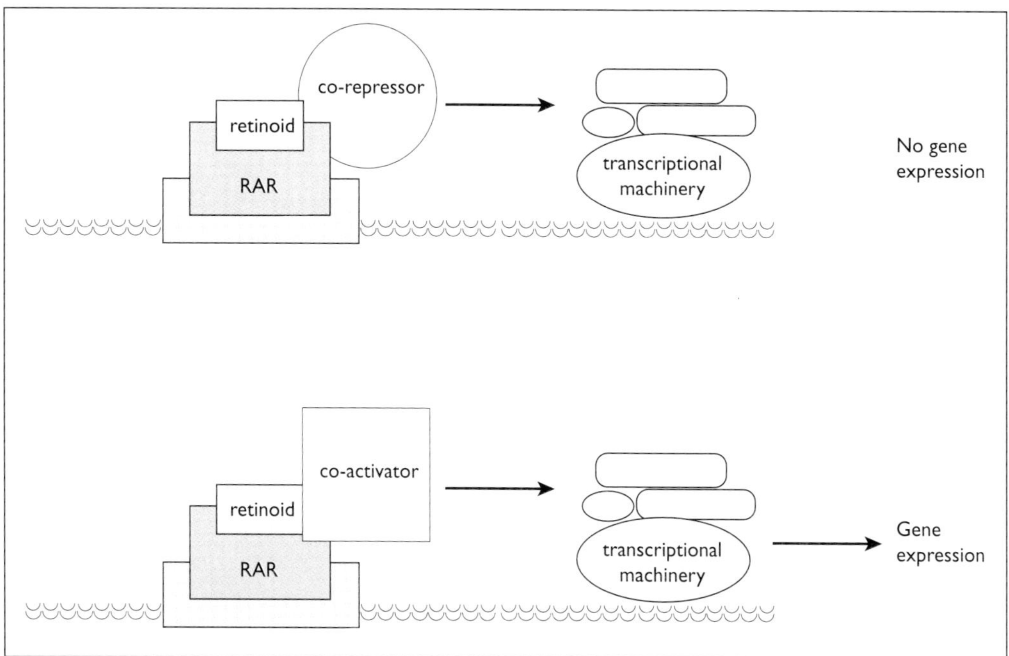

Figure 3.4

Schematic representation of functional consequences of RAR/co-repressor and RAR/co-activator interactions.

good thing, a permanently activated nuclear receptor is physiologically unacceptable, and there has to be an equilibrium process by which the ligand is released from the receptor.

The second intriguing question is: how does this shape change involving movement of helix 12 lead to receptor activation? It appears that the re-positioning of helix 12 over the ligand-binding pocket completes a surface that constitutes the hormone-dependent transactivation function (see above) of the E region of the receptor. This newly completed receptor surface must enable the receptor to contact other proteins involved with the transcriptional machinery and thereby activate transcription. In keeping with this type of mechanism, recent research has resulted in the identification of several accessory proteins that bind differentially with receptors depending on whether or not they are occupied by the ligand. Some of these proteins interact with the nuclear receptor when the receptor is occupied by an agonist, and are called co-activator proteins. Examples of co-activator proteins are CREB-binding protein (CBP) and the related protein SRC-1,[22] which binds to RAR in the presence of RA, as well as receptor-interacting protein 140 (RIP 140),[23] which binds to the oestrogen receptor in the presence of oestrogen. Other proteins, such as nuclear receptor co-repressor (N-CoR)[24,25] and silencing mediator for retinoid and thyroid receptors (SMRT),[26] interact with RAR only in the absence of agonist, and are called co-repressors. Binding of RA to RAR leads to dissociation of the co-repressors, N-CoR and SMRT, from the RAR. Thus, in simple terms, the way in which RA or other agonists activate transcription from RARs appears to be by stabilizing RAR interaction with co-activators and destabilizing interaction with co-repressors. Presumably the co-activators provide a positive 'communication link' between RARs and the transcriptional machinery, while the co-repressors prevent this communication (Figure 3.4).

Therapeutic opportunity within complexity

The current state of knowledge about retinoid receptors provides a picture of great complexity: multiple receptors, multiple dimerization permutations, different response elements and a variety of accessory proteins. However, within this complexity lie new and significant therapeutic opportunities. The therapeutic uses and the many limitations of the currently available retinoids are well documented. These retinoids are of great value in the treatment of acne, psoriasis and other dermatoses, as well as some cancers such as acute promyelocytic leukaemia.[27] Their clinical use is, however, complicated by many toxic side-effects, including mucocutaneous, lipid, bone and CNS toxicities, and teratogenicity. We hypothesize that therapeutic efficacy in specific diseases as well as individual toxicities are mediated by different receptors. The basic goal of our research is to identify retinoid ligands that activate only those receptors and functions that are pertinent to efficacy in a given disease in the hope that the therapeutic use of such compounds will be accompanied by attenuated toxicity.

In our research, we have asked questions such as: can one make ligands that bind to one receptor subtype and not to others? Can different ligands cause different shape changes in a receptor? What are the functional consequences of these different shape changes? As a first step in achieving receptor and function selectivity, we have made compounds that are specific for the RAR family[28] or RXR family.[29,30] We have also made compounds that are completely specific for the RAR-α subtype.[31] Our preliminary data indicate that these selective compounds do indeed have much more restricted pharmacological actions, and also do not exhibit some of the classical retinoid toxicities. Of particular interest was a series of compounds that bound with high affinity to the RARs but did not activate transcription from the receptors.[32] In fact, these compounds are potent and effective antagonists of transcriptional activity induced by RA and other RAR agonists. These RAR antagonists effectively block retinoid-induced toxicities in vivo, suggesting that they can be used clinically for the treatment and prevention of mucocutaneous toxicity produced by systemic retinoids such as isotretinoin (Accutane).[33] These molecules have a bulky substituent group at carbon 1 of the retinoid skeleton. We speculate that this substituent prevents helix 12 from closing completely over the ligand-binding pocket and thereby preventing the hormone-dependent transactivation function from forming. Thus the mouse is still attracted to the trap, but the trap can no longer be completely sprung. It is therefore possible to make a retinoid that induces an RAR shape or conformation that is different from that induced by the natural hormone, RA.

As discussed above, one functional consequence of unusual receptor conformations induced by novel ligands is the lack of gene transcriptional activation and hence the ability of such ligands to act as antagonists. This implies that RAR antagonists will destabilize RAR/co-activator interactions and possibly stabilize RAR/co-repressor interactions. Our preliminary investigations indicate that this is indeed the case. These results suggested that the simple model of RAR activation shown in Figure 3.4 should be modified. In the enhanced model (Figure 3.5), an RAR has a certain amount of basal gene transcriptional activity in the absence of any ligand and this basal activity is dependent on an equilibrium among RARs, co-activators and co-repressors. It is entirely possible that a co-activator and a co-repressor molecule can bind to RAR at the same time. In fact, this type of equilibrium situation is the more likely scenario in vivo, where the relative stoichiometries of RARs and intermediary proteins will be different depending on the cell type. An agonist that stabilizes RAR/co-activator interaction and destabilizes RAR/co-repessor interaction shifts the equilibrium towards more bound co-activator, and hence causes an increase over basal gene transcriptional activity. A ligand that binds to RAR and does not cause a conformational change in the receptor, or causes a conformational change that is ineffectual in changing the RAR/co-activator/co-repressor equilibrium of the unbound receptor, will not change basal gene transcriptional activity. However, these compounds, which we call neutral antagonists, can block the activity of an agonist by competing for binding to RAR. Based on our revised model shown in Figure 3.5, we hypothesized that it would be possible to devise molecules that would stabilize RAR/co-repressor interactions and concomitantly destabilize RAR/co-activator interactions and shift the equilibrium towards more co-repressor-bound RARs, and that such molecules would actually decrease the basal level of gene transcriptional activity. We have termed such molecules inverse agonists, since they do the exact opposite of agonists. It is indeed possible to design such molecules, and we have shown that the classical RAR 'antagonists' that bind to receptor but do not activate transcription can be divided into two classes: neutral antagonists, which do not change the basal activity of RARs, and inverse agonists, which decrease the basal activity.[34] Such RAR inverse agonists are a completely novel class of retinoids, and their biology remains undefined. Our current research efforts are directed towards unraveling this biology and discovering therapeutic applications for this unique class of compounds.

Another activity of retinoid receptors that is of great therapeutic importance is their ability to antagonize other nuclear transcription factors.[12] Of these transcription factors, one of the most studied is AP-1, a dimer of the proteins c-Jun and c-Fos that is up-regulated in a variety of inflammatory and proliferative diseases. AP-1 induces several genes that are important in inflammatory and hyperproliferative pathways, and the ability of retinoids to

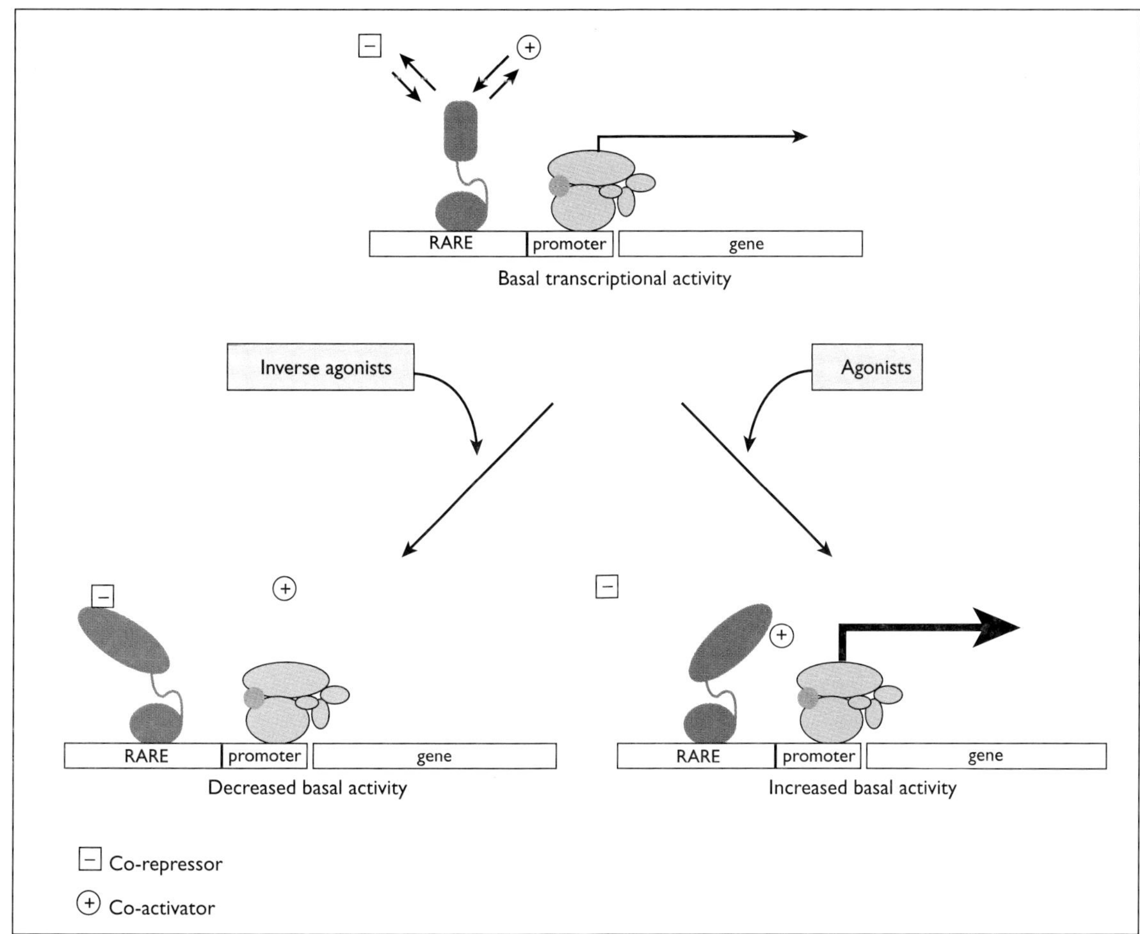

Figure 3.5

Equilibrium model of RAR transcriptional activation.

antagonize the activities of AP-1 and related transcription factors appears to be critical for their anti-inflammatory and anti-proliferative properties. Recent research has suggested that the molecular basis of this antagonism is that RARs and transcription factors such as AP-1 share common co-activator proteins.[22] Thus an agonist will enhance binding of a common co-activator to RAR, sequestering it away from AP-1 and thereby antagonizing AP-1-induced gene transcription. A corollary of this effect is that RAR-mediated gene transcription is also increased. Since anti-AP-1 effects are important for some of the therapeutic effects of retinoids, particularly their anti-inflammatory and anti-proliferative effects, and since some of the toxic effects of retinoids undoubtedly stem from their transcriptional activation effects, it may be useful to separate the anti-AP-1 effect of retinoids from their gene-transcriptional effects. The question then is: can RAR be induced to adopt a shape in which it interacts strongly with co-activator yet orients the latter in a manner that will not activate gene-transcription? We[35] and others[36] have shown that this is possible by demonstrating that the anti-AP-1 and transactivation properties of retinoids are separable with the use of appropriate retinoid ligands. Another interesting question is whether RARs can 'cross-talk' with other members of the steroid/retinoid nuclear receptor superfamily? The molecular basis for such cross-talk would be commonly shared intermediary proteins in a manner analogous to that observed for RAR/AP-1 interactions. Thus if RAR and another nuclear receptor shared a common co-activator that was present in limiting quantities in a given cell, then an RAR agonist can antagonize the activity of the other nuclear receptor by competing away the required co-activator. Conversely, if a common co-repressor was shared between RAR and the other nuclear receptors then an RAR inverse agonist will be able to potentiate the gene-transcriptional activity of this receptor by sequestering co-repressor. Examples of this type of nuclear receptor cross-talk have been observed,[37] but the phenomenon has not been extensively investigated.

The importance of retinoids as mediators of fundamental physiological functions has been recognized for several decades. Several retinoids have also been used successfully in clinical medicine, particularly in dermatology. However, a comprehensive understanding of how these powerful compounds work at the molecular level has become possible only after the discovery of the nuclear retinoid receptors in the late 1980s. The details of the molecular mechanisms of action of retinoids at the receptor level are being worked out only now. Only by a deep and thorough understanding of these molecular mechanisms will the undoubtedly vast therapeutic potential of retinoids be fully realized. The reality is that the very power of retinoids, which stems from the breadth and depth of their biological actions, is actually self-limiting in terms of clinical applications. The development of highly efficacious retinoids with much lower toxicity will require the exploitation of the fine nuances of retinoid receptor/intermediary protein/response elements interactions with receptor- and function-selective retinoids.

References

1. Wolbach SB, Howe PR, Tissue changes following deprivation of fat-soluble A vitamin. *J Exp Med* (1925) **43**: 753–77.
2. Wolbach SB, Howe PR, Epithelial repair in recovery from vitamin A deficiency. *J Exp Med* (1933) **57**: 511–26.
3. Wald G, The biochemistry of vision. *Annu Rev Biochem* (1953) **22**: 497–526.
4. Rando RR, Polyenes and vision. *Chem Biol* (1996) **3**: 255–62.
5. Petkovich M, Brand NJ, Krust A, Chambon P, A human retinoic acid receptor which belongs to the family of nuclear receptors. *Nature* (1987) **330**: 444–50.
6. Giguere V, Ong, ES, Segui, P, Evans, RM, Identification of a receptor for the morphogen retinoic acid. *Nature* (1987) **330**: 624–9.
7. Mangelsdorf DJ, Umeseno K, Evans RM, The retinoid receptors. In: Sporn MB, Roberts AB, Goodman DS (eds). *The retinoids: Biology, chemistry, and medicine.* Raven Press: New York, 1994, Vol 8, pp 319–49.
8. Mangelsdorf DJ, Ong ES, Dyck JA, Evans RM, Nuclear receptor that identifies a novel retinoic acid response pathway. *Nature* (1990) **345**: 224–9.
9. Levin AA, Sturzenbecker LJ, Kazmer S et al, 9-*cis* Retinoic acid stereoisomer binds and activates the nuclear receptor RXRα. *Nature* (1992) **355**: 359–61.
10. Heyman RA, Mangelsdorf DJ, Dyck JA et al, 9-*cis* Retinoic acid is a high-affinity ligand for the retinoid X receptor. *Cell* (1992) **68**: 1–20.
11. Fisher GJ, Talwar HS, Xiao JH et al, Immunological identification and functional quantitation of retinoic acid and retinoid X receptor proteins in human skin. *J Biol Chem* (1994) **269**: 20629–35.

12. Nagpal S, Chandraratna RAS, Retinoids as anti-cancer agents. *Current Pharmaceutical Design* (1996) **2**: 295–316.
13. Yu VC, Delsert C, Andersen B et al, RXRβ: a coregulator that enhances binding of retinoic acid, thyroid hormone, and vitamin D receptors to their cognate response elements. *Cell* (1991) **67**: 1251–66.
14. Zhang X-K, Lehmann J, Hoffman B et al, Homodimer formation of retinoid X receptor induced by 9-*cis* retinoic acid. *Nature* (1992) **358**: 587–91.
15. Roy B, Taneja R, Cahmbon P, Synergistic activation of retinoid acid (RA)-responsive genes and induction of embryonal carcinoma cell differentiation by an RA receptor α (RARα)-, RARβ-, or RARγ-selective ligand in combination with a retinoid X receptor-specific ligand. *Mol Cell Biol* (1995) **15**: 6481–7.
16. Rosen ED, O'Donnell AL, Koenig RJ, Ligand-dependent synergy of thyroid hormone and retinoid X receptors. *J Biol Chem* (1992) **267**: 22010–13.
17. Perlmann T, Rangarajan PN, Umesono K, Evans RM, Determinants for selective RAR and TR recognition of direct repeat HREs. *Genes Dev* (1993) **7**: 1411–22.
18. Umesono K, Murakami KK, Thompson CC, Evans RM, Direct repeats as selective response elements for the thyroid hormone, retinoic acid, and vitamin D_3 receptors. *Cell* (1991) **65**: 1255–66.
19. Bourguet W, Ruff M, Chambon P et al, Crystal structure of the ligand-binding domain of the human nucleur receptor RXRα. *Nature* (1995) **375**: 377–82.
20. Renaud JP, Rochel N, Ruff M et al, Crystal structure of the RARγ ligand-binding domain bound to all-*trans* retinoic acid. *Nature* (1995) **378**: 681–9.
21. Wagner RL, Aprilett JW, McGrath ME et al, A structural role for hormone in the thyroid hormone receptor. *Nature* (1995) **378**: 690–7.
22. Kamei Y, Xu L, Heinzel T et al, A CBP integrator complex mediates transcriptional activation and AP-1 inhibition by nuclear receptors. *Cell* (1996) **85**: 403–14.
23. Cavailles V, Danvois S, L'Horset F et al, Nuclear factor RIP140 modulates transcriptional activation by the estrogen receptor. *EMBO J* (1995) **14**: 3741–51.
24. Horlein AJ, Naar AM, Heinzel T, Ligand-independent repression by the thyroid hormone receptor mediated by a nuclear receptor co-repressor. *Nature* (1995) **377**: 397–404.
25. Kurokawa R, Soderstrom M, Horlein A et al, Polarity specific activities of retinoic acid receptors determined by a co-repressor. *Nature* (1995) **377**: 451–4.
26. Chen JD, Evans RM, A transcriptional co-repressor that interacts with nuclear hormone receptors. *Nature* (1995) **377**: 454–7.
27. Meng-er H, Yu-chen Y, Shu-rong C et al, Use of all-*trans*-retinoic acid in the treatment of acute promyelocytic leukemia. *Blood* (1988) **72**: 567–72.
28. Chandraratna RAS, Gillett SJ, Song TK et al, Synthesis and pharmacological activity of conformationally restricted, acetylenic retinoid analogs. *Bioorg Med Chem Lett* (1995) **5**: 523–7.
29. Beard RL, Chandraratna RAS, Colon DF et al, Synthesis and structure-activity relationships of stilbene retinoid analogs substituted with heteroaromatic carboxylic acids. *J Med Chem* (1995) **38**: 2820–9.
30. Vuligonda V, Lin Y, Chandraratana RAS, Synthesis of highly potent RXR-specific retinoids: the use of a cyclopropyl group as a double bond isostere. *Bioorg Med Chem Lett* (1996) **6**: 213–8.
31. Teng M, Duong TT, Klein ES et al, Identification of a retinoic acid receptor α subtype specific agonist. *J Med Chem* (1996) **39**: 3035–8.
32. Johnson AJ, Klein ES, Gillett SJ et al, Synthesis and characterization of a highly potent and effective antagonist of retinoic acid receptors *J Med Chem* (1996) **38**: 4764–7.
33. Standeven AM, Johnson AT, Escobar M, Chandraratna RAS, Specific antagonist of retinoid toxicity in mice. *Toxicol Appl Pharmacol* (1996) **138**: 169–75.
34. Klein ES, Pino ME, Johnson AT et al, Identification and functional separation of retinoic acid receptor neutral antagonists and inverse agonists. *J Biol Chem* (1996) **271**: 22692–6.
35. Nagpal S, Athanikar J, Chandraratna RAS, Separation of transactivation and AP1 antagonism functions of retinoic acid receptor a. *J Biol Chem* (1995) **270**: 923–7.

36. Fanjul A, Dawson MI, Hobbs PD et al, A new class of retinoids with selective inhibition of AP-1 inhibits proliferation. *Nature* (1994) **372**: 107–11.

37. Casanova J, Hebner E, Selmi-Ruby S et al, Functional evidence for ligand-dependent dissociation of thyroid hormone and retinoic acid receptors from an inhibitory cellular factor. *Mol Cell Biol* (1994) **14**: 5756–65.

4 Pharmacokinetics of oral retinoids in clinical practice

Anders Vahlquist, Ola Rollman and Braham Shroot

Introduction

Correct clinical use of oral synthetic retinoids requires some knowledge of the pharmacology and pharmacokinetics of the drugs. For example, disregarding the fact that etretinate persists in the blood for several years after cessation of medication may prove disastrous for female patients who plan to become pregnant. Another example of clinical relevance is the importance of taking the drugs together with food in order to optimize their absorption and thus improve the cost–benefit ratio of the treatment.

Virtually all retinoids share the following pharmacological and chemical characteristics: they are more or less hydrophobic compounds, tightly bound to plasma proteins, are chemically unstable in the presence of oxidizing compounds and ultraviolet radiation, and have comparatively long elimination half-lifes. As a group, oral retinoids thus have little in common with other drugs.

The following review of retinoid pharmacokinetics emphasizes clinically important aspects of their usage such as dosage regimens, interactions with other drugs and precautions in patients with hepatic or renal dysfunction. Apart from 9-cis retinoic acid only oral retinoids which are on the market (isotretinoin, etretinate and acitretin) or are in routine use for non-dermatological indications (tretinoin) will be discussed. For a more comprehensive survey, the reader is referred to references 1–6.

Isotretinoin

Isotretinoin (13-*cis*-retinoic acid) is closely related chemically to natural vitamin A (Table 4.1) and should possibly be considered to be a member of the group of endogenous compounds resulting from vitamin A metabolism, since trace amounts of the compound are present in normal human plasma. The origin and biological function of this retinoid under physiological conditions is not yet clear but 13-*cis*-isomerization from all-*trans*-retinoic acid has been suggested to occur in vivo.[7]

Absorption

After ingestion in its usual clinical dosage form (dissolved in oil contained in a soft elastic gelatin capsule) isotretinoin (Roaccutane,

Table 4.1 **Main pharmacokinetic properties of currently available oral retinoids**

	Vitamin A	*Isotretinoin*	*Etretinate*	*Acitretin*
Configuration				
Ring	β-Ionone	β-Ionone	Monoaromatic	Monoaromatic
Side-chain	All-*trans*	13-*cis*	All-*trans*	All-*trans*
End group	Alcohol or fatty acyl ester	Acid	Ethyl ester	Acid
Molecular weight	286	300	354	326
Therapeutic dosage range (mg/kg per day)	0.2–2	0.5–2	0.5–1.0	0.3–0.75
Main carrier in plasma	RBP or lipoproteins	Albumin	Lipoproteins	Albumin
Estimated oral availability (%)	50–80	21–25	30–70	36–95
Storage sites				
Liver	Yes	No	No	No
Fat	(Yes)	No	Yes	No
Adrenals	(Yes)	Not known	Yes	(No)
Terminal elimination half-life	75–250 days	10–20 h	100–150 days	50–60 h***
Active metabolites	Retinal and retinoic acid	Retinoic acid?	Acitretin Isoacitretin?	Isoacitretin? Etretinate***
Average tissue levels* (ng/g)				
Epidermis	250	75	150**	50
Dermis	200	Not known	175	Not known
Subcutis	2000	<30	≥5000	100
Sebaceous glands	1000	~50	Not known	Not known

*In patients receiving 0.5–0.8 mg/kg per day of the drug for at least 1 month (data from refs 16, 18, 44, 45, 64 and 69, and the authors' unpublished observations).
**Sum of parent compound and main metabolite.
***Dependent on whether reverse metabolism to etretinate occurs or not (see text)

Accutane) slowly dissolves in the gastrointestinal fluid and is then rapidly absorbed from the gut. Accordingly, a lag period of 0.5–2 h follows ingestion of the drug until it appears in the general circulation.[8,9]

The absolute oral availability of isotretinoin has not been established, as disposition data following administration in humans are not available. Results obtained in animal studies, however, indicate that 21–25 per cent of an oral dose, when administered under fasting conditions, will reach the general circulation in parent compound form.[1,10] The low availability is probably due to extensive presystemic biodegradation in the gut lumen, incomplete absorption and first-pass hepatic clearance of the drug.[10]

In common with other lipid-soluble compounds, the absorption of isotretinoin is enhanced when administered with food. Accordingly, the relative oral availability was found to be approximately 1.5–2 times greater

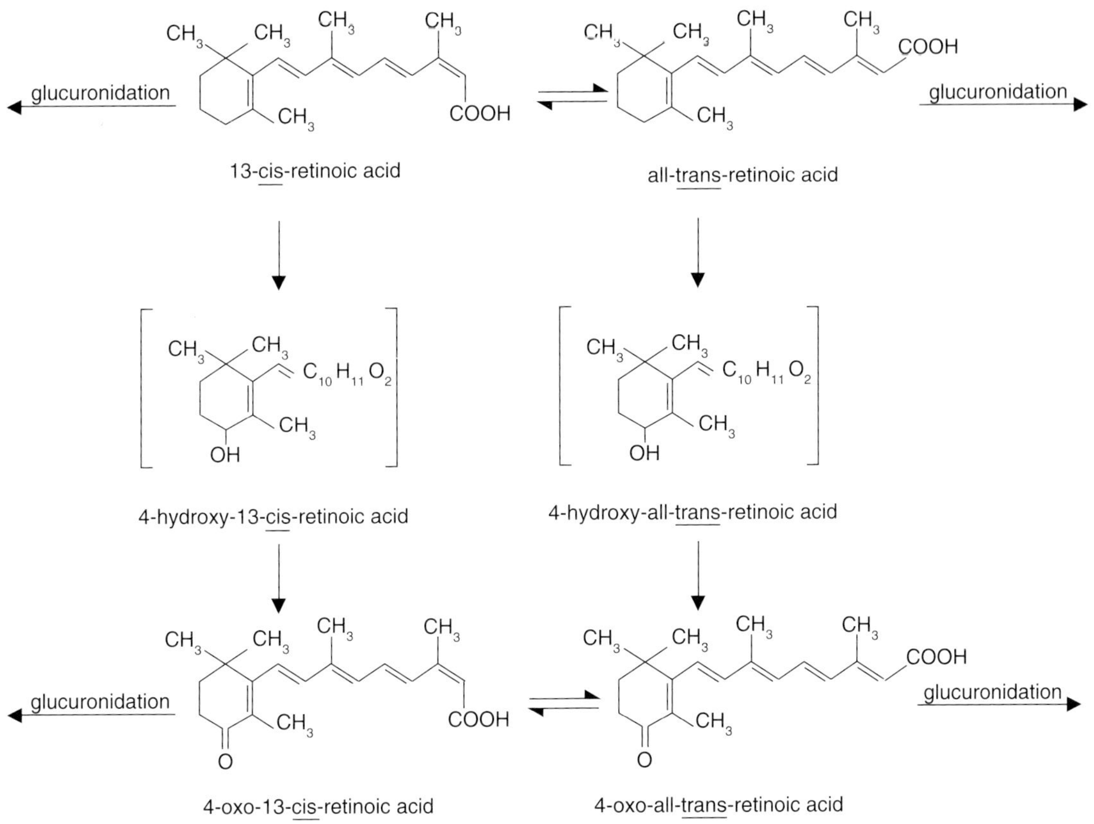

Figure 4.1

Main metabolites of isotretinoin in humans.[1]

when the dose was taken with breakfast rather than with water.[11] The potentiating effect of food on isotretinoin absorption also occurs when the drug is taken either 1 h before or 1 h after the meal. The mechanism of the food–drug interaction, and which food components are of decisive importance, is not yet clear, but factors such as increased drug solubility in the gut lumen, delayed gastric emptying and stimulated bile flow may facilitate drug absorption.

Metabolism and excretion

The hepatic metabolism of isotretinoin is extensive and involves oxidation of the cyclohexinyl ring, glucuronide conjugations and, possibly, isomerization of the polyene side chain.[12] The principal metabolic pathways suggested are two parallel routes, as shown in Figure 4.1. Isotretinoin is converted to 4-oxo-isotretinoin, with the 4-hydroxy metabolite postulated as being an intermediate reaction product. Additional metabolites identified in human bile include glucuronide conjugates of 16- and 18-hydroxy-isotretinoin. Other hepatic metabolites are likely to be formed, but have not yet been fully characterized chemically.[12]

The all-*trans* isomer of retinoic acid represents a plausible metabolite of high biological potency. The appearance in plasma of the all-*trans*-retinoic acid close to threshold levels has been observed following a single dose of isotretinoin,[8,13] with the proportion of the all-*trans* isomer increasing to as much as 10–20 per cent of the plasma isotretinoin concentration during long-term retinoid therapy.[14] Although representing a true pharmacological reaction, the absolute extent of isomerization of isotretinoin in vivo is difficult to determine, since acidic retinoids are extremely susceptible to artificial isomerization during sample storage and analysis.

Isotretinoin is rapidly eliminated by the liver and kidneys, with the main mechanism of excretion being hepatic clearance. Both the unmodified drug and oxidized metabolites are conjugated with glucuronic acid in the liver prior to biliary excretion. Negligible amounts of isotretinoin appear unmodified in the bile,[12] as is generally expected of a lipophilic drug tightly bound to plasma proteins. The kidney is a less important site of excretion with little 4-oxo-isotretinoin and virtually no parent drug being identified in urine.[6,8]

Blood concentration – time profiles of isotretinoin

In a single-dose study where 80 mg isotretinoin (0.9–1.2 mg/kg) was given to a group of ten acne patients, a wide range of peak drug levels (98–535 ng/ml blood; mean, 262 ng/ml) was attained 2–4 h after taking the drug.[15] The areas under the blood concentration–time curves (AUC) ranged from 0.9 to 4.6 μg·h/ml (Figure 4.2a). The great inter-patient variability in isotretinoin kinetics can probably be explained by irregular intestinal absorption during fasting conditions, and by enterohepatic recycling, as suggested by the appearance of secondary or tertiary plasma drug peaks in some patients.[9,15]

On subsequent multiple dosing (40 mg twice daily) of the same group of acne patients, steady-state conditions were attained in 5–7 days with predose drug levels (mean, 160 ng/ml blood) and AUC (mean, 3.1 μg·h/ml) displaying considerable differences among patients, although remaining at a fairly constant day-to-day level in an individual patient (Figure 4.2b,c). Likewise, the rate of disappearance of the drug from blood varied almost four-fold ($t_{1/2}$, 6–22 h) between patients; yet the average $t_{1/2}$ (15 h) in the group of patients did not differ from that following a single dose. Hence, there was no evidence of accumulation or significant change in the pharmacokinetic handling of the drug during long-term retinoid administration in acne patients.

The main metabolite, 4-oxo-isotretinoin, thought to be a pharmacologically inactive by-product,[12] is the predominant drug metabolite present in plasma during repeated dosing. At steady-state, this compound is found in plasma at levels three to four times as high as those of the parent compound. 4-oxo-isotretinoin accumulates slightly during long-term treatment and clears more slowly ($t_{1/2}$, 17–50 h; mean 25 h) from the circulation than does the native drug.[15] A minor proportion of this metabolite is present in blood in its all-*trans* form, 4-oxo-retinoic acid.[13,15]

Plasma protein binding

The transport of isotretinoin is effected almost entirely by albumin leaving only 0.1 per cent of the total drug unbound in plasma.[6] The unbound fraction is constant over the drug's therapeutic concentration range, with no displacement occurring by its metabolites.[1]

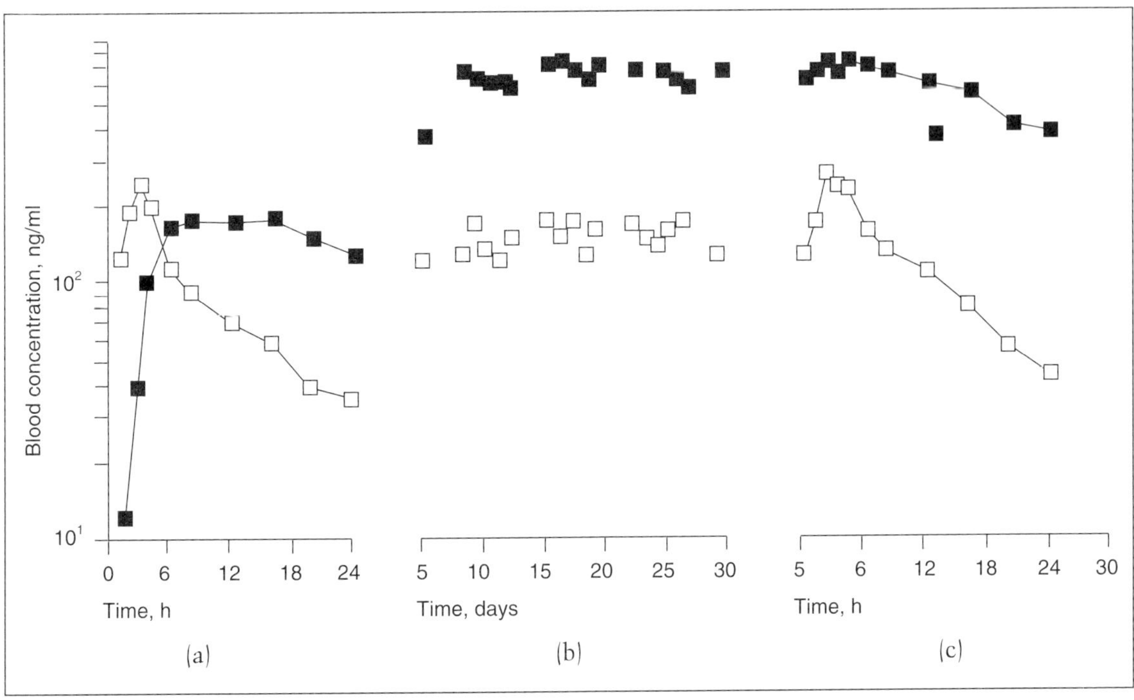

Figure 4.2

Plasma concentration–time profiles of isotretinoin (open squares) and its main metabolite 4-oxo-isotretinoin (closed squares) following single- and multiple-dose administration of oral isotretinoin to acne patients. Mean blood concentrations in ten acne patients **(a)** after a single 80-mg dose, **(b)** during 25 days of 40 mg twice daily dosing, and **(c)** after a final 80-mg dose of isotretinoin.[1,15]

Generally, the unbound, rather than the bound, fraction of a drug is believed to be the one more closely connected with the pharmacological effects of the drug, but no such relationship has been investigated for isotretinoin. Under ordinary therapeutic conditions, plasma albumin is present in a 100-fold molar excess of isotretinoin. Thus only a minute proportion of available binding sites on albumin are occupied by the drug.

There is no evidence to suggest that isotretinoin utilizes or interferes with the transfer mechanism for natural vitamin A in humans.[14,16] Interference with other drugs is discussed below.

Distribution

Once absorbed, isotretinoin is rapidly and widely delivered to the body tissues. The bulk of the drug within the tissues is probably not free, but closely associated with tissue molecules. Experimental studies indicate that proteins are likely to be the predominant binding component for isotretinoin in the skin, whereas lipids seem to play a marginal role.[17]

The tissue distribution of oral isotretinoin in humans has not been studied, except that steady-state drug concentrations in the skin have been determined in acne patients.[16]

During chronic isotretinoin dosing (0.75 mg/kg per day), drug levels in the epidermis (60–120 ng/g wet weight) are generally lower than in the general circulation and comparable to those attained by ordinary doses of etretinate (see Table 4.1). The main metabolite of isotretinoin predominates over the parent drug in the epidermis, reflecting the situation in the plasma. There is no progressive accumulation of the drug in the skin during long-term administration and, in contrast to the more lipid-soluble etretinate, isotretinoin is not stored or retained in the subcutaneous fat. Moreover, analysis of microdissected sebaceous glands from isotretinoin-treated acne patients has shown that the drug is taken up by the target tissue even though present at somewhat higher concentrations in the skin compartments surrounding the sebaceous glands.[18] The metabolic fate of isotretinoin in the pilosebaceous apparatus is not known, but the fact that the drug is not detected in surface sebum collected during oral therapy[19] indicates that extensive metabolism or degradation may take place in the sebocytes or, following drug sequestration, in the follicular epithelium or in the sebum itself. After stopping isotretinoin therapy, drug concentrations in the sebaceous glands decline and no detectable retinoid remains 3 weeks after ceasing medication.[18] Hence, isotretinoin is not specifically deposited or retained in the glands to such an extent as to explain its sustained anti-acne activity.

Placental and breast milk transfer

Epidemiological studies in humans have clearly shown that fetal exposure to therapeutic doses of isotretinoin is associated with an increased risk of major congenital malformations and of miscarriage.[20] Before initiating isotretinoin therapy in a fertile woman, pregnancy must therefore be excluded and a safe contraceptive method practised for 1 month before treatment is begun and throughout the treatment course. After cessation of therapy, contraceptive precautions should be continued to allow plasma drug concentrations to fall below teratogenic levels. Since the critical maternal drug concentration necessary to induce fetal abnormalities in humans is not known, the minimum safe interval between stopping the drug and conception has not been established. Calculating using a half-life twice as long as the average for isotretinoin, the plasma drug concentration (parent compound plus main metabolite) at 2 weeks after discontinuation of treatment ought to be approximately twice the total plasma-concentration of endogenous all-*trans*-retinoic acid, 13-*cis*-retinoic acid and 13-*cis*-4-oxo-retinoic acid (3–6 ng/ml). After another 2-week period off therapy, the estimated drug level should closely approach the physiological concentrations of these acidic retinoids. For kinetic reasons, therefore, it seems advisable to avoid pregnancy for at least 1 month after drug discontinuation. In confirmation, no increased risk of fetal malformation or miscarriage has yet been reported in women adhering to this currently recommended contraceptive advice.[23]

The transplacental transport mechanisms of isotretinoin have not been revealed in humans. Recently, investigation of a 4-month-old fetus aborted by a woman who took isotretinoin during the first trimester showed that 4-oxo-isotretinoin had accumulated in the liver and that low concentrations of the parent drug and metabolite were present in the brain of the fetus.[24] In another report, the drug content was investigated in a 1-month-old embryo from a woman who had unintentionally taken 40 mg isotretinoin daily from the first week of gestation.[25] In the whole embryo, low concentrations of the 4-oxo metabolite were detected, whereas considerable amounts of the parent drug (1.2 µg/g) were found. Notably, even higher concentrations of all-*trans*-retinoic acid (2.8 µg/g) were found in the embryo, supporting the view that the transplacental transfer occurs much more readily with the all-*trans* isomer than the 13-*cis* isomer of retinoic acid.[25,26]

The possible excretion of isotretinoin into human breast milk has not been investigated but is likely to occur, in view of the lipophilic nature of the drug and the known passage of acitretin into mature breast milk.[27] Because of the toxicity of isotretinoin, breast-feeding should be avoided by women taking isotretinoin.

Influence of systemic disease

A small number of post-transplant kidney recipients with mild renal dysfunction (serum creatinine, 170–250 μmol/l) have taken low-dose isotretinoin (0.2–0.5 mg/kg per day) with good anti-acne effect and no clinical signs of retinoid toxicity or deterioration of renal function.[28–30] Similarly, a uraemic patient undergoing haemodialysis was given the full dose of isotretinoin as acne treatment with no evidence of abnormal drug side-effects.[31] Acne patients exhibiting other systemic diseases including diabetes mellitus, ulcerative colitis, epilepsy and multiple sclerosis have safely received ordinary doses of isotretinoin.[32,33]

Interaction with other treatments

Reduced efficacy of isotretinoin therapy has been observed during heavy alcohol intake.[34]

Isotretinoin is metabolized by cytochrome P450 enzymes which are inducible by ethanol and inhibited by, for example, ketoconazole. Increased blood levels of isotretinoin may therefore be expected when the drug is combined with imidazole fungistatics.

Female patients undergoing isotretinoin therapy frequently use combined oral contraceptive steroids. Clinical studies in such patients have not revealed any interaction of isotretinoin with plasma hormone levels or effects of such steroids.[35]

The absorption of fat soluble vitamins may generally be impaired by cholestyramine, broad-spectrum antibiotics, laxatives and antacids containing aluminium and magnesium. Whether these drugs interfere with isotretinoin absorption is, however, not known.

Salicylic acid, indomethacin, phenylbutazone and other acidic drugs with high affinity for albumin, when present in the blood at high therapeutic concentrations, may possibly displace isotretinoin from its protein-binding sites, thereby increasing the unbound fraction of the drug in the plasma.[36] Hypothetically, if co-administered with isotretinoin, such drugs might increase the risk of retinoid toxicity. No such drug interactions, however, have been reported to have occurred in clinical practice.

In a heart transplant recipient treated with cyclosporin, the additional administration of isotretinoin did not significantly affect cyclosporin blood levels.[37] However, detailed kinetic studies on the effect of cyclosporin and isotretinoin combination therapy are lacking.

Carbamazepine pharmacokinetics changed in a patient who took concurrent isotretinoin; plasma levels of the carbamazepine and its main metabolite were decreased.[38] It was suggested that carbamazepine levels should be closely monitored during concurrent isotretinoin therapy in order to avoid inadequate control of epilepsy.

Haloperidol disposition was affected in animals by concurrent isotretinoin administration,[39] but clinically relevant interactions between these drugs have not been reported to have occurred in humans.

Oral tetracycline therapy is not known to interfere with isotretinoin pharmacokinetics but, in common with retinoids, may cause increased intracranial pressure. Its combination with isotretinoin should therefore be avoided.

Drugs considered safe when administered with isotretinoin include penicillin, erythromycin, clindamycin, paracetamol and insulin.[32,33] Since vitamin A and the synthetic retinoids produce additive toxic effects, vitamin A supplementation should be avoided in patients receiving isotretinoin therapy.

Drug interference at the target site by topical dermatological agents has not been investigated. Ultraviolet irradiation may possibly cause physical destruction or isomerization of isotretinoin while present in the skin, since an animal study has shown that both photochemical isomerization and destruction of orally administered isotretinoin take place in the epidermis in vivo.[40]

Interaction with natural vitamin A

Isotretinoin cannot be converted to retinol in vivo, and plasma vitamin A concentrations are not affected by systemic isotretinoin administration.[14,16,41] In contrast, experimental studies indicate that retinoid compounds may interfere markedly with vitamin A-metabolizing enzymes present in the gut, liver, eye and skin. Thus both intestinal retinal reduction and hepatic retinol esterification are inhibited by isotretinoin in vitro.[42] It is not known to what extent these interactions affect the absorption or hepatic storage of natural vitamin A in patients taking the drug. In peripheral tissues, however, isotretinoin therapy may cause clinically relevant interactions such as abnormal night vision.[43] Also, oral isotretinoin is known to interfere with vitamin A levels in human skin.[16] In acne patients given isotretinoin at a daily dosage of 0.5–1 mg/kg for 3–6 months the epidermal and sebaceous gland contents of vitamin A (retinol including its esters) increased by at least 50–100 per cent. In contrast, the cutaneous concentrations of 3,4-dehydroretinol (vitamin A_2), an endogenous metabolite of retinol,[44] decreased to almost undetectable levels. These effects probably involve metabolic interference of isotretinoin on vitamin A metabolism in the target tissue. The retinol concentration is low in acne lesions and dehydroretinol accumulates in hyperproliferative skin disorders,[45] so their modification with isotretinoin may have therapeutic implications. Future studies on the metabolism and biological effects of retinoids at the cellular level are required to clarify the importance of drug–vitamin A interactions during isotretinoin therapy.

Summary and practical advice

The human pharmacology of isotretinoin has been investigated in appropriate target populations, i.e. patients having nodulocystic acne or severe disorders of keratinization. The pharmacokinetic profile of oral isotretinoin in these disease states is similar to that observed in healthy subjects, and is less complex than that of etretinate. The disposition of isotretinoin is not modified by repeated dosing and does not involve accumulation, delayed elimination or biotransformation to a main active metabolite. Only a small and variable proportion of the drug can gain access to the general circulation owing to presystemic losses. The intestinal absorption will improve significantly if the drug is taken with food, and for reasons of availability, convenience and compliance it is recommended that the retinoid be taken once or twice daily with a meal. Concomitant vitamin A therapy should be avoided, and other drugs or disease states that may affect the absorption, protein binding, hepatic metabolism and excretion of isotretinoin should be considered carefully when prescribing this drug. The teratogenicity of retinoids requires effective contraceptive measures to be taken in women of childbearing age. Fortunately, the clearance of isotretinoin is rapid enough to permit conception 1 month after discontinuation of isotretinoin therapy.

During routine drug monitoring the positive and undesirable clinical effects are evaluated during therapy. A correlation between clinical response and drug concentrations in plasma, skin or the pilosebaceous apparatus should be expected, but has yet not been proved. Sensitive and specific high-performance liquid chromatography techniques enable therapeutic concentrations of isotretinoin and its metabolites to be determined in plasma or target tissues.[16,46–48] The application of these techniques may prove valuable in future studies on skin pharmacology of retinoids and in certain therapeutic situations, e.g. in clinical dose–response studies, in matters of drug failure, toxicity or compliance, and in disease states that may critically affect isotretinoin pharmacokinetics.

Aromatic retinoids – etretinate and acitretin

To this family of retinoids belong compounds which have an aromatic (as opposed to a β-ionone) ring structure. These so-called second generation (monoaromatic) or third generation (polyaromatic) retinoids are new synthetic compounds which do not occur in nature. Only two aromatic retinoids are freely available for oral administration. For practical reasons, etretinate (Tigason, Tegison) and acitretin (etretin, Neotigason, Soriatane) are discussed together.

From both pharmacokinetic and historical viewpoints, etretinate is the prodrug of acitretin (Figure 4.3). Etretinate is the ethyl ester of acitretin and probably lacks biological activity per se (owing to a blocked carboxy terminus). However, etretinate was selected for initial clinical trials because animal experiments indicated that it was absorbed better from the gastrointestinal tract than acitretin. Only later did it become clear that both drugs are equally well absorbed in humans.

Absorption

The average oral availability of etretinate is 40 per cent, with a large interindividual variation of 30–70 per cent, and that of acitretin is 59 per cent (range 36–95 per cent).[49,50] Absorption takes place mainly in the jejunum, and patients with severe malabsorption (e.g. owing to intestinal resection) may require increased dosage of the drugs. Unfortunately, no parenteral formulations are available for use in these situations.

Following oral administration of etretinate and acitretin, peak plasma concentrations of unmodified drug are reached within 4 h. By ingesting the drugs together with fat-containing food, the maximum plasma concentration and overall bioavailability of the drugs are approximately twice as high as under fasting conditions.[51,52] However, the rate of absorption and formation of metabolite are unaffected. Plasma concentrations of etretinate were three- to five-fold higher with a fat-rich meal of whole milk, but were unchanged with a high-carbohydrate meal, as compared with administration during a complete fast.[51] A likely explanation for this observation is that fat-stimulated bile secretion enhances solubility and intestinal absorption of the drug via the lymphatics.

Metabolism and excretion

Figure 4.3 shows the metabolic pathways of etretinate and acitretin in humans. Conversion of etretinate to acitretin begins during absorption and continues after the drug has been absorbed, but is never complete. Because transport from the gut proceeds mainly via the lymphatics, first-pass metabolism in the liver is minimal.

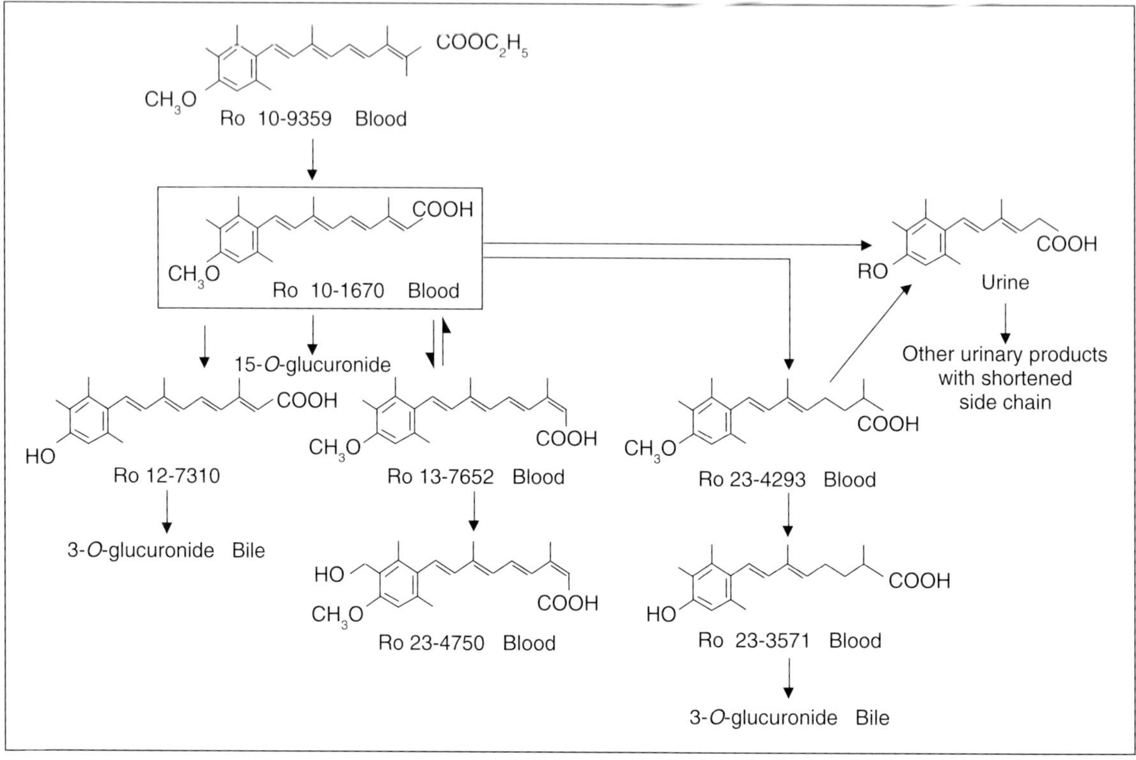

Figure 4.3

Main metabolites of etretinate (Ro 10-9359) and acitretin (Ro 10-1670) in humans.[49]

Back metabolism of acitretin

The initial hopes for acitretin relied on an assumption that the drug would be rapidly excreted after discontinuation of therapy. However, recent studies have revealed that acitretin is partly metabolized by esterification to etretinate-like metabolites that are lipid bound and may persist for variable times after drug discontinuation.[53–56] Conversion of acitretin to etretinate seems to be facilitated by ethanol ingestion.[55] In this report ten patients were treated with 30 mg of acitretin daily for 3 months. Seven patients had detectable levels of plasma etretinate between 2.5 and 56.7 ng/ml. All seven patients had consumed ethanol. However, back metabolism to etretinate may also occur in patients who deny ethanol consumption.[55]

Oxidation of aromatic retinoids requires cytochrome P450 and is thus amenable to enzyme induction, for instance by alcohol and barbiturates.

Acitretin appears to be eliminated exclusively by metabolism, with the resultant metabolites excreted to an equal extent by the hepatic and renal routes. Virtually no unmodified drug or isoacitretin is found in the urine or the bile.[49]

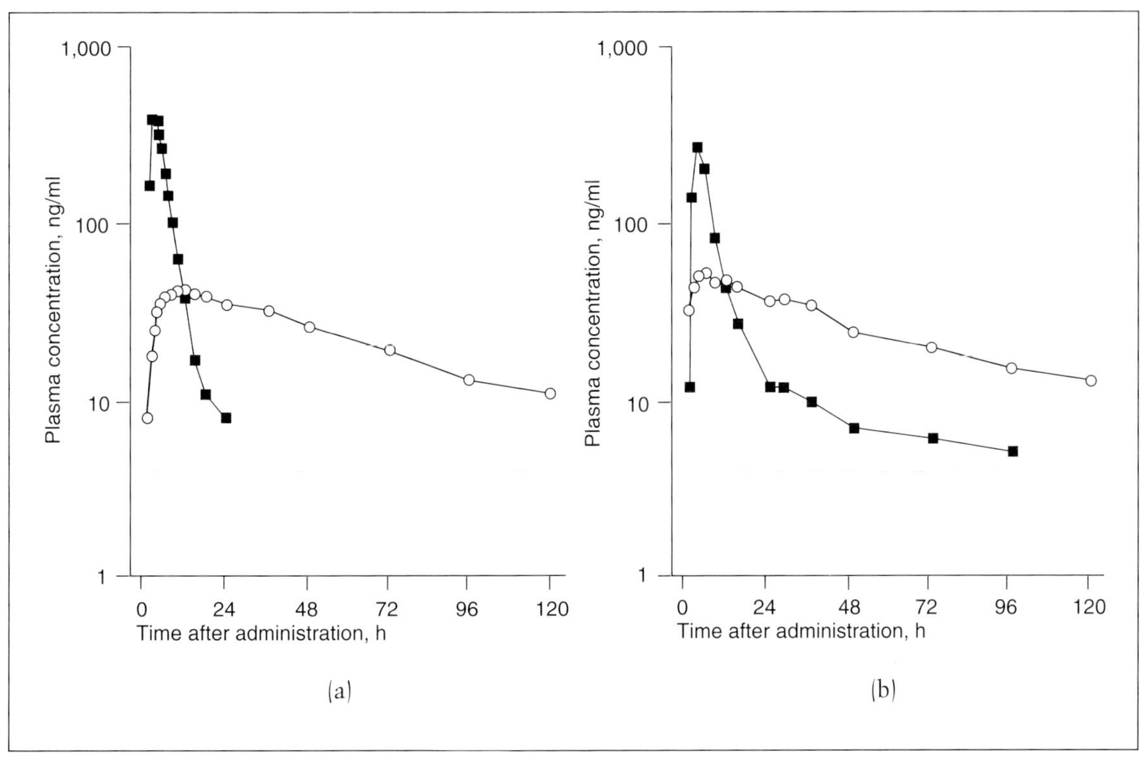

Figure 4.4

Plasma concentration–time profile of acitretin (closed squares) and its main metabolite isoacitretin (13-*cis*-acitretin, open circles) following **(a)** single and **(b)** multiple-dose administrations of oral acitretin (50 mg once daily) to a group of healthy subjects (mean values are shown).[49]

Instead, metabolites with shortened side chains predominate and, at least in the bile, these metabolites are to a large extent conjugated with glucuronic acid.[57]

Blood concentration–time profiles of aromatic retinoids

Plasma concentrations of unchanged drug and metabolites appear to be characterized by linear pharmacokinetics following ascending single and multiple doses of acitretin and etretinate, that is, increasing the dose of the drugs results in predictable increases in concentration of the parent compounds and metabolites in plasma.[49,58–60] Following multiple dosing of etretinate (50 mg once daily), predose steady-state concentrations of unmodified drug, acitretin and 13-*cis*-acitretin (isoacetretin) averaged 100, 40 and 170 ng/ml, respectively.[49] When acitretin was given as parent drug in the same dosage (50 mg) the corresponding values were on average 20 ng/mg (acitretin) and 100 ng/ml (13-*cis* acitretin).[49,59]

Typical pharmacokinetic profiles of acitretin are shown in Figure 4.4. The most conspicuous feature is the rapid appearance of isoacitretin in plasma. The concentration–time curve of the isomer is quite different from that of the unchanged drug, with a half-life about 1.5-fold higher than that of acitretin. Steady-state trough plasma concentrations ($C_{ss,min}$) of both compounds are reached within 7–10 days, which is consistent with the elimination half-life of the two retinoids. During chronic therapy the predosing level of 13-*cis*-acitretin is usually some 3–5-fold higher than for acitretin. The terminal elimination of acitretin (given as parent drug) is shorter as compared to etretinate; after multiple-dose administration for 3 months a terminal half-life of 50–60 h has been found.[49,60] Occasionally, the half-life is longer (see above).

The multiple-dose kinetics of etretinate, on the other hand, are not predictable from the single-dose data. Thus, apparent half-life increases from approximately 7 h after a single dose to 120 days during chronic therapy.[4,61–63] In line with this, steady-state conditions will usually take 20–30 days to become established. The long terminal half-life of etretinate is explained by a slow leakage of the drug from the fat tissues.[64] Low levels (<2 ng/ml) of etretinate and its metabolite acitretin can frequently be demonstrated in plasma for more than 2 years after stopping etretinate therapy.[65] Occasionally, the half-life may be significantly longer, and in one patient etretinate was still present at a level of 46 ng/ml even at day 500 post-therapy.[66]

Pharmacokinetics and age, body weight and gender

Plasma concentrations of unmodified drug and 13-*cis*-acitretin tended to be greater in the elderly than in young healthy volunteers,[67] but in 57 patients undergoing acitretin therapy no significant correlation was found between age and steady-state drug concentrations.[49] It should be emphasized, however, that no pharmacokinetic data are available for children or for the very old. In one study (Hoffmann–La Roche, data on file) no significant correlation was found between total plasma drug concentrations at steady state and the body weight of patients undergoing therapy with acitretin. Comparable information on the relationship between the pharmacokinetics of etretinate and age, body weight and gender is not available. However, in patients with larger amounts of body fat, etretinate tends to have an increased elimination half-life.[66]

Plasma protein binding

Etretinate and acitretin are up to 99.9 per cent protein bound in plasma. This implies that variations in binding protein concentrations and competition with other drugs that are tightly bound to plasma proteins can affect the pharmacokinetics of these aromatic retinoids. Etretinate binds both to the lipoproteins and to albumin, whilst acitretin (and presumably isoacitretin as well) is bound almost exclusively to albumin.[68] Retinol-binding protein, the natural carrier of vitamin A, plays little if any role in the transport of synthetic retinoids. The delivery of drug to the cells is thought to occur via the free fraction not bound to plasma proteins, but an interesting possibility is that lipoprotein-bound etretinate may also enter cells directly via receptors for low and very low-density lipoproteins.

Distribution

Both etretinate and acitretin bind tightly to tissue proteins and become widely distributed throughout the body. The distribution volumes of acitretin and etretinate have been estimated to about 3.5 l/kg and 40 l/kg, respectively, in humans.[63] The high value for

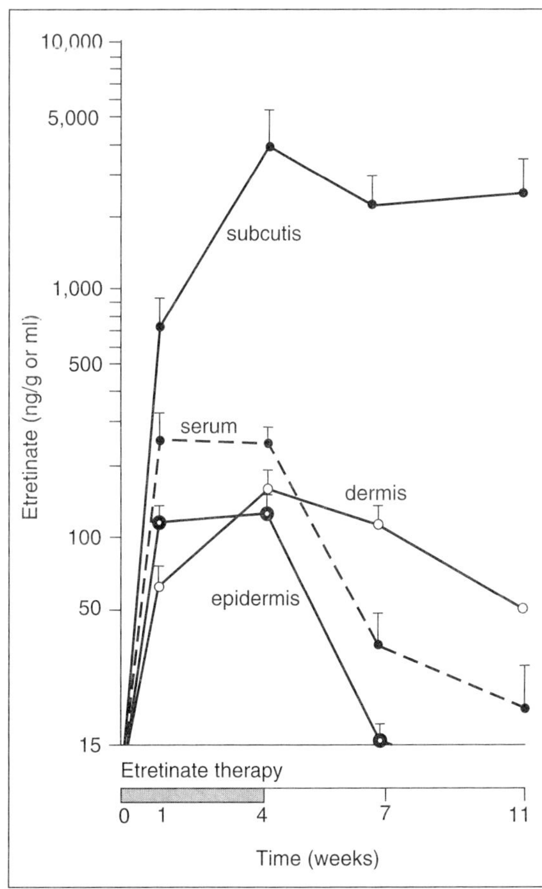

Figure 4.5

Tissue distribution of etretinate in epidermis, dermis and subcutis during long-term etretinate therapy.[64] The values represent the sum of native drug and main metabolite concentrations.

etretinate is consistent with an extensive accumulation in the tissues. High-affinity sites for etretinate are fat tissue and the adrenals, but not the liver as might be expected from its structural relationship to vitamin A.[69] Accumulation in fat explains the very long biological half-life of etretinate. Thus within a few weeks of starting therapy, the etretinate concentration in fat is almost 100-fold that in most other tissues (Figure 4.5). Later, the fat tissues appear to become saturated and during long-term therapy about 50–100 mg of etretinate is stored in the fat.[64] There is reason to believe that obese individuals have a greater distribution volume for etretinate than lean individuals, whereas the distribution volume for acitretin is independent of body weight. Nothing is known about the mobilization of etretinate from adipose tissues in situations of starvation and major fat catabolism.

A matter of great concern is whether acitretin treatment of a patient previously exposed to etretinate retards the elimination of the latter drug from fat tissue. If this were the case, the terminal half-life of etretinate in plasma would rise to values exceeding the average of 120 days and this would have to be taken into consideration, for example, when giving contraceptive advice to women after stopping sequential etretinate and acitretin treatment. However, there are some preliminary data suggesting that this is not a great problem.[66]

Etretinate concentrations in liver and other non-adipose tissues are in the range 100–1500 ng/g.[64,69] However, if fatty degeneration of the liver is present, hepatic concentrations of etretinate may attain higher values.[70] The total drug concentration in the epidermis averages 150 ng/g during chronic dosing (50 mg daily) and does not change with time, in contrast to the concentration in adipose tissue (Figure 4.5).[64] The drug disappears fairly rapidly from the epidermis, a finding consistent with the rapid reversal of mucocutaneous side-effects after stopping treatment.

The tissue distribution of acitretin has been less assiduously studied. In a preliminary report, Laugier et al[71] found about 200 ng/g and 50 ng/g, of acitretin and isoacitretin, respectively, in full-thickness skin biopsies from psoriasis patients receiving 30 mg of acitretin daily. We found considerably lower levels (20–50 ng/g) of acitretin in epidermis from similarly treated patients.[54] Acitretin is usually absent from the adipose tissue but metabolic products may be present at concentrations of about 1000 ng/g.[54]

In separate skin distribution studies, acitretin was given by the oral route[72] or applied topically.[73] Steady-state plasma levels were reached after 10 days following an oral dose of 50 mg/day. The all-*trans*- and 13-*cis*-acitretin isomers were quantified using sensitive and precise procedures for assay in plasma, suction blister fluid and skin tissue, obtained by punch biopsy, shave biopsy or suction blister roofs. Drug concentrations were determined following a single 24-h application of a saturated solution of acitretin in isopropyl myristate. Adequate skin concentrations were found when the drug was delivered by either route (>160 ng/g tissue); none the less, acitretin is not effective in psoriasis, when applied topically. These observations give rise to speculation concerning target cell and gradient concentrations in the skin. Essentially, it remains to be shown that sustained levels in the dermis/upper epidermis (as shown above, Figure 4.5) are established, when the drug is applied topically.

Placental and breast milk transfer

The aromatic retinoids are teratogenic in humans and in other animals. The drugs must therefore somehow be conveyed from mother to fetus. Although little is known about the passage to the offspring it seems to occur via the placenta. Etretinate concentrations in amniotic fluid were below detection limit[74] in a woman who became pregnant 9 months after stopping treatment when her plasma drug level was approximately 10 ng/ml. Acitretin (and probably etretinate) is also transferred via breast milk, but it may be calculated that an infant would receive less than 50 μg/day of the drug if breast-fed by an acitretin-treated mother.[27] Although the oral dose thus received by a suckling infant would correspond to only 1.5 per cent of the maternal dose level, the toxic potential of the retinoid justifies its avoidance in breast-feeding women.

Teratogenic levels of acitretin

Although the minimal level at which acitretin is teratogenic is unknown, conception, it was hoped, could safely occur within a short time (1 or 2 months) after acitretin was discontinued without any subsequent risk of teratogenicity. However, because of the re-esterification of acitretin (see above), recommendations for 2 years' post-acitretin contraception have generally been adopted in those countries where acitretin is approved for prescription (as of October 1996, acitretin has not been approved by the US Food and Drug Administration). An overview of pharmacokinetics and teratogenicity relating to acitretin enables the reader to grasp the key features of a restricted therapeutic use of this oral retinoid in women of childbearing age.[75]

Importantly, the inability to detect plasma etretinate and acitretin was recently questioned as predictor of the absence of these teratogens in the tissues.[76] In this study women were found who had detectable amounts of the drug in fat tissue for up to 29 months post-therapy. Moreover, Maier and Hönigsmann[77] recently reported that acitretin-related material could be demonstrated in the fat tissue for up to 52 months post-therapy, i.e. much longer than the recommended contraception period of 2 years! However, it is still uncertain if low levels of acitretin and etretinate in fat tissue, without detectable amounts of the drug in the blood, are teratogenic.

Influence of systemic disease

In a study of four etretinate-treated patients suffering from psoriasis and chronic renal failure (CRF), the dose requirements, clinical responses and side-effects of the drug were similar to those seen in other psoriasis patients with normal kidney function.[78] Also, the half-life over a 24-h period for etretinate and acitretin (as metabolite) was similar in CRF and control patients, as were the mean trough ($C_{ss, min}$) and peak levels of acitretin. A notable difference, however, was that the plasma levels of unmodified drug were on average twice as high in CRF patients. It is not known whether this indicates a greater bioavailability of etretinate in CRF patients or simply reflects the fact that the hyperlipidaemia frequently observed in these patients facilitates etretinate transport in plasma.

Recently, the pharmacokinetics of acitretin and isoacitretin (as metabolite) were investigated in six patients undergoing haemodialysis.[79] The patients were given 50 mg acitretin. The mean AUC in the CRF patients was about half that in the control subjects. No retinoids were detectable in the dialysate. The investigators suggested that an impaired absorption of acitretin (possibly due to simultaneous intake of aluminium hydroxide) might have accounted for the lower plasma concentrations of acitretin in patients undergoing haemodialysis. Another possibility is that the lower albumin concentrations in patients on dialysis caused an increased volume of distribution owing to a decreased binding to plasma proteins.

Although CRF does not seem to interfere markedly with the elimination of aromatic retinoids, it must be remembered that these patients are intrinsically prone to develop hypervitaminosis A. This is due to a decreased glomerular filtration of retinol-binding protein carrying vitamin A.[80]

Little is known about the pharamacokinetics of aromatic retinoids in hepatic failure. There are anecdotal reports of psoriasis patients with liver cirrhosis being successfully treated with etretinate. In a recent study of etretinate pharmacokinetics in seven psoriasis patients with liver fibrosis, essentially normal plasma levels and half-lives of unchanged drug and metabolites were found.[81] However, there was a six-fold interindividual variation with regard to the systemic availability of etretinate. Three of the patients had manifest cirrhosis but none had severe hepatic failure. Therefore, it cannot be excluded that with increasingly severe failure and eventual hepatic coma the degradative metabolism of the aromatic retinoids will be markedly impaired. A comprehensive review by Grønhøj Larsen provides a useful description of the pharmacokinetics of etretinate and acitretin which includes details of analytical methods.[82]

In psoriasis patients with impaired glucose tolerance, etretinate therapy reduces the endogenous insulin secretion in response to a glucose load.[83] This finding is in agreement with a similar study of acitretin in healthy volunteers[84] and suggests that the aromatic retinoids improve glucose tolerance by increasing the sensitivity to endogenous insulin. To date, no clinical consequences in terms of blood glucose control or antidiabetic therapy have been reported in diabetic patients treated with aromatic retinoids.

Psoriasis may itself affect the pharmacokinetics of etretinate. For unknown reasons the peak plasma levels after a single 75 mg oral dose were lower in psoriatic patients (545 ± 183 ng/ml, n=6) than in control subjects (930 ± 73 ng/ml).[66,78]

Interaction with other treatments

General considerations about co-administration of aromatic retinoids with oral contraceptive agents, antibiotics, fat-soluble vitamins, etc. appear to be the same as noted above for isotretinoin. Some examples are listed below.

Phenytoin displaces etretinate in vitro but there are no reports of significant interaction problems in clinical practice. In one patient on continuous phenytoin therapy, a 3-month course of therapy with etretinate 25 mg twice daily did not affect the plasma level of phenytion, and the response to etretinate was apparently unaffected (Vahlquist, unpublished observation). In contrast, therapy with primidone (Mylepsin), another type of anticonvulsive agent, reportedly made a patient resistant to etretinate therapy.[85] Although the mechanism of this interaction is not known, primidone is known to stimulate the oxidative catabolism of many other drugs. Similarly, carbamazepine reduced the responsiveness to etretinate in one patient.[86]

The safety of concurrent methotrexate and etretinate/acitretin therapy has been questioned.[87] Etretinate treatment (30 mg daily) raised the methotrexate level after a 10-mg infusion to twice the pre-treatment value in one patient.[88] Similarly, in a study of six patients, significantly higher methotrexate levels (mean about 30 per cent higher) were found in those receiving concurrent etretinate therapy.[89] These data only refer to parenteral use of methotrexate. Absorption and disposition rates of etretinate during combined treatment with methotrexate were not significantly altered compared with previous data in psoriatic patients receiving only etretinate.

Combined treatment with immunosuppressive agents is occasionally used but no data are available concerning possible pharmacokinetic interactions with the aromatic retinoids. Concurrent administration of azathioprine and prednisolone in kidney-transplanted individuals does not, however, significantly change the dose–response or side-effect profile of etretinate.[90] It could be argued that cyclosporin, which is a highly lipid-soluble drug, might interact with etretinate at the level of absorption and tissue disposition, but no such interactions between the two drugs have yet been reported. However, since both drugs are metabolized by cytochrome P450 isoenzymes, it has been suggested that the increased blood levels of cyclosporin found in a psoriatic patient were due to metabolic interaction from co-administered etretinate.[91] The hypothesis was supported by in vitro data, but another study failed to demonstrate any effect of etretinate on human liver cyclosporin metabolism.[92] As discussed for isotretinoin, drugs like ketoconazole and liarozole, which inhibit cytochrome P450, may possibly impede the metabolic degradation of aromatic retinoids too. There is a theoretical risk for interaction also with gemfibrozil (a lipid-lowering agent), although this was not a clinical problem when acitretin and gemfibrozil were used together in a recent study.[93]

A clinically important interaction was recently reported with warfarin.[94] A patient with skin lymphoma who received warfarin and, subsequently, etretinate required an increased warfarin dosage. It was suggested in this case that etretinate induced the hepatic metabolism of warfarin. Thus, careful monitoring of anticoagulant activity is essential in warfarin-treated patients who receive retinoids. By contrast, phenprocoumon does not seem to interact with acitretin.[95]

Combination with PUVA therapy did not affect the concentrations of acitretin in plasma but the pharmacokinetic profile of 13-*cis*-acitretin was changed (50 per cent increase in AUC).[96] Conversely, taking etretinate does not alter the pharmacokinetics of psoralen (8-MOP) and should not require any change in PUVA treatment.[97] Although animal experiments indicate that UV irradiation promotes 13-*cis* isomerization of acitretin in skin and blood, the total drug concentration in the skin appears to be unaffected by irradiation.[40,64]

In contrast to isotretinoin, the aromatic retinoids do not affect the concentrations of vitamin A in tissue.[45,64]

Summary and practical advice

Etretinate is a prodrug of acitretin with a molecular weight about 10 per cent higher than acitretin. Thus equimolar dosage of the two drugs means a 10 per cent lower dose by weight of acitretin. The daily doses, usually 30–75 mg etretinate or 20–50 mg acitretin, can be given as either a single or split dose. To improve treatment efficacy, and to reduce costs, patients should be recommended to take the drugs with the main meal of the day.

Three compounds must be considered in the pharmacokinetics of etretinate: the unchanged drug, acitretin and isoacitretin. Metabolic degradation seems to take place both in the liver and in the extrahepatic tissues. Excretion of metabolites occurs via both urine and bile. Virtually no unchanged drug is excreted. Marked abnormalities in the plasma concentrations of albumin and lipoproteins may affect the plasma and tissue concentrations of the drugs. Furthermore, compounds such as phenytoin, verapamil and other lipophilic drugs may displace (or be displaced by) the aromatic retinoids.

The interindividual variations in the plasma concentrations of the drugs following oral administration of acitretin and etretinate appear to be partly related to incomplete absorption. However, interindividual variations in the plasma concentrations are not critical in the treatment of patients since the dose is adjusted to individual response. Although diurnal variations in the plasma concentration of the drugs may be directly reflected in the tissues,[6,71,72] clinical effects and mucocutaneous side-effects appear to be independent of whether the daily dose of the drug is given once or is divided.

Storage in fat explains the much longer biological half-life of etretinate (as parent drug or metabolite of acitretin) compared with acitretin. Obese patients retain more etretinate than lean patients but the length of therapy (over 2 months) will not markedly influence the amount of drug stored. Storage of etretinate in fat (and the adrenals) does not appear to cause any other untoward effects, but with regard to its slow elimination and teratogenicity, fertile women should maintain effective contraception for at least 2 years after cessation of etretinate or acitretin therapy. Kidney and liver diseases are not absolute contraindications for treatment with aromatic retinoids, but the risk of aggravating a liver disease with a toxic drug hepatitis must be considered. In the case of uraemia the potential addition of retinoid toxicity to a pre-existing hypervitaminosis A should alert the clinician when patients develop characteristic side-effects. Monitoring of the plasma concentrations of the drugs and metabolites is recommended when the dose–response is abnormal.

Tretinoin

All-*trans*-retinoic acid induces leukaemic cell differentiation and oral administration of this drug results in remission in a high proportion of patients with acute promyelocytic leukemia (APL). However, remissions tend to be brief, and pharmacokinetic studies in patients have shown that this may be explained by an accelerated clearance from the plasma, during the 6-week treatment period. A dose of 45 mg/m^2 per day was given as a single dose on the first day, and as two divided doses thereafter. A plasma half-life value of 0.8 ± 0.1 h was calculated with peak plasma levels of 347 ± 266 ng/ml being reached 1–2 h after drug ingestion.[98]

Compared with isotretinoin, tretinoin is more rapidly cleared from plasma (1 h as compared with 13 h), minimal conversion from all-*trans* to 13-*cis*-RA is observed in the plasma, and less of the corresponding 4-oxo metabolite is accumulated with the all-*trans* isomer than with the 13-*cis* isomer. It appears that tretinoin can induce its own catabolism.[99]

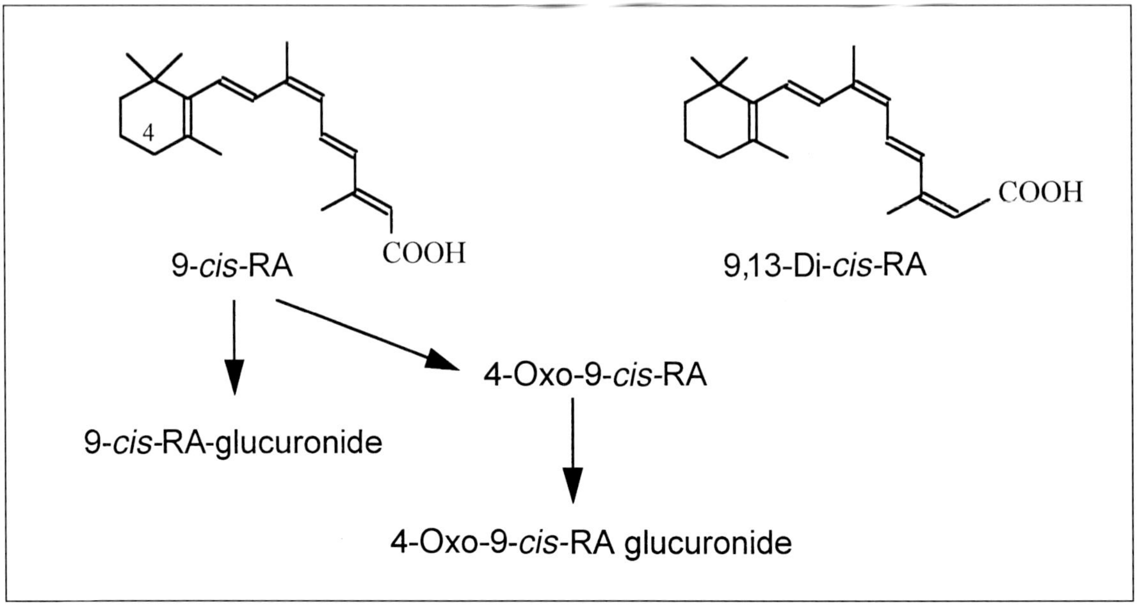

4
COOH
9-*cis*-RA
COOH
9,13-Di-*cis*-RA
4-Oxo-9-*cis*-RA
9-*cis*-RA-glucuronide
4-Oxo-9-*cis*-RA glucuronide

Figure 4.6

Main metabolites of 9-*cis*-retinoic acid in humans.[103]

These factors may explain why a significant cohort of APL patients acquire retinoid resistance. To overcome this, ketoconazole ingested orally (200 mg/day) 1 h prior to RA administration increased the area under the plasma drug concentration-time curve (AUC) from approximately 250 ng/h per ml to 300 ng/h per ml. Interindividual variability is very high, and patients would have to be carefully preselected (fast/slow RA catabolizers) for these combination regimens.

Intermittent administration of all-*trans*-RA (7 days on/7 days off, 40 mg/m^2), gave rise to relatively consistent plasma exposures of about 150 μM/l per min at the beginning of each cycle.[100]

However, pharmacokinetic considerations alone do not explain reduced efficacy of RA. Oral low dose tretinoin (from 30 to 10 ng/day) produced satisfactory therapeutic results in patients with oral and cutaneous forms of lichen planus.[101]

9-cis-*Retinoic acid*

Another naturally occuring retinoid, showing promise in cancer therapy, 9-*cis*-retinoic acid possesses similar plasma pharmacokinetic properties to all-*trans*-retinoic acid. After repeat doses of ≥140 mg/m^2, AUC values were reduced to more than 50 per cent relative to day 1 values. Plasma half-life values ranged from 1 to 2 h (compare all-*trans*-RA). Very little all-trans or 13-cis-retinoic acid could be detected.[102]

Two hours following the last of 28 daily doses of 9-*cis*-retinoic acid (20 mg/day), a metabolic profile study revealed that, in plasma, the major metabolites appear to be 4-oxo-retinoic acid (isomer mixture) (Figures 4.1 and 4.6) and 9,13-di-*cis*-RA (or retinoic acid) (Figure 4.6). In the urine evidence of glucuronidation was found, whereas in faeces mainly unchanged drug was found, implying poor oral absorption. Future human studies will no doubt help select effective treatment regimens.[103]

Conclusion

The contents of this chapter show that, as a drug class, retinoids are far from optimal in terms of providing easy choices for oral therapy. Low efficacy, poor absorption, high inter-individual variation or long residence time limits the use of existing drugs. They are all, however, based on similar chemical templates, and it is to be hoped that, in the next decade, major advances will be made with targeted formulations or novel chemical entities.

References

1. Brazzell RK, Colburn WA, Pharmacokinetics of the retinoids isotretinoin and etreinate. *J Am Acad Dermatol* (1982) **6**(4): 643–51.
2. Lambert WE, Meyer E, De Leenheer AP et al, Pharmacokinetics of acitretin. *Acta Derm Venereol (Stockh)* (1994) **S186**: 122–3.
3. Peck GL, Di Giovanna JJ, Synthetic retinoids in dermatology. In: Sporn MB, Roberts AB, Goodman DS (eds). *The retinoids: biology, chemistry and medicine*, 2nd edn. Raven Press: NY, 1994 pp. 631–58.
4. Allen JG, Bloxham DP, The pharmacology and pharmacokinetics of the retinoids. *Pharmacol Ther* (1989) **40**(1): 1–27.
5. Blaner WS, Olson JA, Retinol and retinoic acid metabolism. In: Sporn MB, Roberts AB, Goodman DS (eds). *The retinoids: biology, chemistry and medicine*, 2nd edn. Raven Press: New York, 1994: pp. 229–55.
6. Lucek RW, Colburn WA, Clinical pharmacokinetics of the retinoids. *Clin Pharmacokinet* (1985) **10**: 38–62.
7. Tang G, Russell RM, 13-*cis*-Retinoic acid is an endogenous compound in human serum. *J Lipid Res* (1990) **31**: 175–82.
8. Besner J-G, Leclaire R, Band P et al, Single-dose pharmacokinetic study of 13-*cis*-retinoic acid in man. *Cancer Treat Rev* (1985) **69**(3): 275–7.
9. Khoo K-C, Reik D, Colburn WA, Pharmacokinetics of isotretinoin following a single oral dose. *J Clin Pharmacol* (1982) **22**: 395–402.
10. Cotler S, Buggé CJL, Colburn WA, Role of gut contents, intestinal wall, and liver on the first pass metabolism and absolute bioavailability of isotretinoin in the dog. *Drug Metab Dispos* (1983) **11**(5): 458–62.
11. Colburn WA, Gibson DM, Wiens RE et al, Food increases the bioavailability of isotretinoin. *J Clin Pharmacol* (1983) **23**(11–12): 534–9.
12. Vane FM, Buggé CJL, Rodriguez LC et al, Human biliary metabolites of isotretinoin: identification, quantification, synthesis, and biological activity. *Xenobiotica* (1990) **20**(2): 193–207.
13. Vane FM, Buggé CJL, Identification of 4-oxo-isotretinoin as the major metabolite of 13-*cis*-retinoic acid in human blood. *Fed Proc* (1980) **39**: 757.
14. Goodman GE, Eispahr JG, Alberts DS et al, Pharmacokinetics of 13-*cis*-retinoic acid in patients with advanced cancer. *Cancer Res* (1982) **42**: 2087–91.
15. Brazzell RK, Vane FM, Ehmann CW et al, Pharmacokinetics of isotretinoin during repetitive dosing to patients. *Eur J Clin Pharmacol* (1983) **24**: 695–702.
16. Rollman O, Vahlquist A, Oral isotretinoin (13-*cis*-retinoic acid) therapy in severe acne: drug and vitamin A concentrations in serum and skin. *J Invest Dermatol* (1986) **86**(4): 384–9.
17. Walter K, Kurz H, Binding of drugs to human skin: influencing factors and the role of tissue lipids. *J Pharm Pharmacol* (1988) **40**(10): 689–93.

18. Vahlquist A, Rollman O, Holland DB et al, Isotretinoin treatment of severe acne affects the endogenous concentration of vitamin A in sebaceous glands. *J Invest Dermatol* (1990) **94**: 496–8.
19. Vane MF, Chari SS, Shapiro SS et al, Comparison of the plasma and sebum concentrations of the arotinoid Ro 15-0778 and isotretinoin in acne patients. In: Marks R, Plewig G (eds). *Acne and related disorders*. Martin Dunitz: London, 1989, pp 183–90.
20. Rosa FW, Teratogenicity of isotretinoin. *Lancet* (1983) **ii**: 513.
21. De Leenheer AP, Lambert WE, Claeys I, All-*trans*-retinoic acid: measurement of reference values in normal human serum by high performance liquid chromatography. *J Lipid Res* (1982) **23**: 1362–7.
22. Eckhoff C, Nau H, Identification and quantitation of all-*trans*- and 13-*cis*-retinoic acid and 13-*cis*-4-oxoretinoic acid in human plasma. *J Lipid Res* (1990) **31**(8): 1445–54.
23. Dai WS, Hsu M-A, Itri LM, Safety of pregnancy after discontinuation of isotretinoin. *Arch Dermatol* (1989) **125**: 362–5.
24. Benifla JL, Ville Y, Imbert MC, Fryman R, Thomas A, Pons JC, Fetal tissue dosages of retinoids. Experimental study concerning a case of isotretinoin (Roaccutan) administration and pregnancy. *Fetal Diagn Ther* (1995) **10**(3): 189–91.
25. Creech-Kraft J, Nau H, Embryonic retinoid concentrations after material intake of isotretinoin. *N Engl J Med* (1989) **321**: 262.
26. Creech-Kraft J, Kochhar DM, Scott WJ et al, Low teratogenicity of 13-*cis*-retinoic acid (isotretinoin) in the mouse corresponds to low embryo concentrations during organogenesis: comparison to the all-*trans* isomer. *Toxicol Appl Pharmacol* (1987) **84**: 474–82.
27. Rollman O, Pihl-Lundin I, Acitretin excretion in human breast milk. *Acta Derm Venereol (Stockh)* (1990) **70**: 487–90.
28. Tam M, Cooper A, The use of isotretinoin in a renal transplant patient with acne. *Br J Dermatol* (1987) **116**: 463.
29. Marcusson JA, Tyden G, Acne conglobata in transplant patients treated with isotretinoin. *Br J Dermatol* (1988) **118**: 310–12.
30. Kiraly C, Valkamo MH, Renal transplantation and isotretinoin. *Acta Derm Venereol (Stockh)* (1990) **70**: 540.
31. Beightler EL, Tyring SK, The use of isotretinoin in a patient undergoing kidney hemodialysis. *J Am Acad Dermatol* (1990) **23**(4): 758.
32. Macdonald Hull S, Cunliffe WJ, The safety of isotretinoin in patients with acne and systemic diseases. *J Dermatol Treat* (1989) **1**: 35–7.
33. Cunliffe WJ (ed.), Side effects of acne therapy. In: *Acne*. Martin Dunitz: London, 1989, pp 288–324.
34. Soria C, Allegue F, Galiana J et al, Decreased isotretinoin efficacy during acute alcohol intake. *Dermatologica* (1991) **182**: 203.
35. Orme M, Back DJ, Cunliffe WJ et al, Isotretinoin and oral contraceptive steroids. *Br J Clin Pharmacol* (1984) **17**(2): 227–8.
36. Rowland M, Tozer T, Interacting drugs. In: *Clinical pharmacokinetics – concepts and applications*. Lea & Febiger: Philadelphia, 1989, pp 255–75.
37. Bunker CB, Rustin MHA, Dowd PM, Isotretinoin treatment of severe acne in post-transplant patients taking cyclosporine. *J Am Acad Dermatol* (1990) **22**(4): 693–4.
38. Marsden JR, Effect of isotretinoin on carbamazepine pharmacokinetics. *Br J Dermatol* (1988) **119**: 403–4.
39. Straw G, Kirch D, Freed WJ, Haloperidol and metabolite concentrations in the rat after concurrent isotretinoin administration: a preliminary report. *Pharmacol Toxicol* (1988) **63**(5): 326–8.
40. Berne B, Rollman O, Vahlquist A, UV-induced isomerization of oral retinoids in vitro and in vivo in hairless mice. *Photodermatol Photoimmunol Photomed* (1990) **7**: 146–52.
41. Kerr IG, Lippman ME, Jenkins J et al, Pharmacology of 13-*cis*-retinoic acid in humans. *Cancer Res* (1982) **42**: 2069–73.
42. Dew SE, Wardlaw SA, Ong DE, Effects of pharmacological retinoids on several vitamin A-metabolizing enzymes. *Cancer Res* (1993) **53**(13): 2965–69.
43. Weleber RG, Denman ST, Hanifin JM, Cunningham WJ, Abnormal retinal function associated with isotretinoin therapy for acne. *Arch Ophthalmol* (1986) **104**: 831–7.

44. Vahlquist A, Vitamin A in human skin: I. detection and identification of retinoids in normal epidermis. *J Invest Dermatol* (1982) **78**: 89–93.
45. Vahlquist A, Törmä H, Rollman O et al, Distribution of natural and synthetic retinoids in the skin. In: Saurat JH (ed). *Retinoids: new trends in research and therapy*. Karger: Basel, 1985, pp 159–67.
46. Furr HC, Barua AB, Olson JA, Analytical Methods. In: Sporn MB, Roberts AB, Goodman DS (eds). *The retinoids: biology, chemistry and medicine*, 2nd edn. Raven Press: 1984, New York, pp 179–210.
47. Vahlquist A, Törmä H, Rollman O, Andersson E, High-performance liquid chromatography of natural and synthetic retinoids in human skin samples. In: Packer L (ed.). *Methods in enzymology. Retinoids Part B, cell differentiation and clinical applications,* vol 190. Academic Press: San Diego, 1990, pp 163–74.
48. Wyss R, Chromatography of retinoids. *J Chromatogr* (1990) **531**: 481–508.
49. Brindley CJ, Overview of recent clinical pharmacokinetic studies with acitretin (Ro 10-1670, etretin). *Dermatologica* (1989) **178**: 79–87.
50. Brindley CJ, Dubach UC, Forgo I, Absolute bioavailability of acitretin (Ro 10-1670). In: Reichert U, Shroot B (eds). *Pharmacology of retinoids in the skin*. 8th CIRD Symposium on Advances in Skin Pharmacology, 1–3 Sept, 1988, Karger: Basel, 1989, pp 207–10.
51. Colburn WA, Gibson DM, Rodriguez LC et al, Effect of meals on the kinetics of etretinate. *J Clin Pharmacol* (1985) **25**: 583–9.
52. McNamara PJ, Jewell RC, Jensen BK et al, Food increases the bioavailability of acitretin. *J Clin Pharmacol* (1988) **28**: 1051–5.
53. Chou R, Wyss R, Huselton C et al, A newly discovered xenobiotic pathway: ethyl ester formation. *Life Sci* (1991) **49**: 169–72.
54. Larsen FG, Vahlquist C, Andersson E et al, Oral acitretin in psoriasis: drug and vitamin A concentrations in plasma, skin and adipose tissue. *Acta Derm Venereol (Stockh)* (1992) **72**: 84–8.
55. Larsen FG, Jakobsen P, Knudsen J et al, Conversion of acitretin to etretinate in psoriatic patients is influenced by ethanol. *J Invest Dermatol* (1993) **100**: 623–7.
56. Meyer E, De Bersaques J, Lambert WE et al, Skin, adipose tissue and plasma levels of acitretin with rare occurrence of esterified acitretin during long-term treatments. *Acta Derm Venereol (Stockh)* (1993) **73**: 113–15.
57. Vane FM, Buggé CJL, Rodriguez LC, Identification of etretinate metabolites in human bile. *Drug Metab Dispos* (1989) **17**: 275–9.
58. Wills RJ, Rodriguez LC, Lin AH et al, Dose-proportional absorption of etretinate after doses of 25, 50, 75 and 100 mg. *Pharm Res* (1987) **4**: 420–4.
59. Gollnick H, Bauer R, Brindley C et al, Acitretin versus etretinate in psoriasis. *J Am Acad Dermatol* (1988) **19**: 458–69.
60. Al-Mallah N, Brindley CJ, Bun H et al, Pharmacokinetics of acitrein (Ro 10-1670) following multiple oral dosing. In: Reichert U, Shroot B (eds). *Pharmacology of retinoids in the skin*. 8th CIRD Symposium on Advances in Skin Pharmacology, 1–3 Sept, 1988. Karger: Basel, 1989, pp 181–7.
61. Massarella J, Vane F, Buggé C et al, Etretinate kinetics during chronic dosing in severe psoriasis. *Clin Pharmacol Ther* (1985) **37**: 439–46.
62. Grønhøj Larsen F, Jakobsen P, Grønhøj Larsen C et al, Single dose pharmacokinetics of etretin and etretinate in psoriasis patients. *Pharmacol Toxicol* (1987) **61**: 85–8.
63. Grønhøj Larsen F, Jakobsen P, Grønhøj Larsen C et al, Pharmacokinetics of etretin and etretinate during long-term treatment of psoriasis patients. *Pharmacol Toxicol* (1988) **62**: 159–65.
64. Rollman O, Vahlquist A, Retinoid concentrations in skin, serum and adipose tissue of patients treated with etretinate. *Br J Dermatol* (1983) **109**: 439–47.
65. DiGiovanna JJ, Zech LA, Ruddel ME et al, Etretinate: persistent serum levels after long-term therapy. *Arch Dermatol* (1989) **125**: 246–51.
66. Lambert WE, De Leenheer AP, De Bersaques JP et al, Persistent etretinate levels in plasma after changing the therapy to acitretin. *Arch Dermatol Res* (1990) **282**: 343–4.
67. Lambert W, De Bersaques J, Brindley CJ et al, Comparison of the pharmacokinetics of acitretin (Ro 10-1670) in young and elderly

subjects. In: Reichert U, Shroot B (eds). *Pharmacology of retinoids in the skin*. 8th CIRD Symposium on Advances in Skin Pharmacology, 1–3 Sept, 1988. Karger: Basel 1989, pp 211–14.

68. Vahlquist A, Michaëlsson G, Kober A et al, Retinoid-binding proteins and the plasma transport of etretinate (Ro 10-9359) in man. In: Orfanos CE et al (eds). *Retinoids. Advances in basic research and therapy*. Springer: Berlin, 1981, pp 109–16.
69. Vahlquist A, Rollman O, Pihl-Lundin I, Tissue distribution of aromatic retinoid (etretinate) in three autopsy cases: drug accumulation in adrenals and fat. *Acta Derm Venereol (Stockh)* (1986) **66**: 431–4.
70. Roenigk HH, Retinoids: effects on the liver. In: Saurat J-P (ed). *Retinoids: new trends in research and therapy*. Karger: Basel, 1985, pp 476–88.
71. Laugier J-P, Berbis P, Brindley C et al, Determination of acitretin and 13-*cis*-acitretin in skin. *Skin Pharmacol* (1989) **2**: 181–6.
72. Laugier JP, Surber C, Bun H et al, Determination of acitretin in the skin, in the suction blister, and in plasma of human volunteers after multiple oral dosing. *J Pharm Sci* (1994) **83**: 623–8.
73. Surber C, Wilhelm KP, Berman D, Maibach HI, In vivo skin penetration of acitretin using three sampling techniques. *Pharm Res* (1993) **10**: 1291–4.
74. Vahlquist A, Rollman O, Etretinate and the risk for teratogenicity: Drug monitoring in a pregnant woman for 9 months after stopping treatment. *Br J Dermatol* (1990) **123**(1): 131.
75. Bouvy ML, Sturkenboom MCJM, Cornel MC, De Jong van den Berg LTW, Stricker BHC, Wesseling H, Acitretin (Neotigason): A review of pharmacokinetics and teratogenicity and hypothesis on metabolic pathways. *Pharm Weekbl Sci Ed* (1992) **14** (2): 33–7.
76. Sturkenbook MCJM, DeJong-van den Berg LTW, van Voorst-Vader PC, Cornel MC, Stricker BHCH, Wesseling H, Inability to detect plasma etretinate and acitretin is a poor predictor of the absence of these teratogens in tissue after stopping acitretin treatment. *Br J Clin Pharmacol* (1994) **38**: 229–35.
77. Maier H, Hönigsmann H, Concentrations of etretinate in plasma and subcutaneous fat after long-term acitretin. *Lancet* (1996) **348**: 1107.
78. Vahlquist A, Etretinate pharmacokinetics in chronic renal failure. A preliminary study in psoriasis patients. *Dermatologica* (1987) **175**: 224–8.
79. Stuck AE, Brindley CJ, Busslinger A et al, Pharmacokinetics of acitretin and its 13-*cis* metabolite in patients on haemodialysis. *Br J Clin Pharmacol* (1989) **27**: 301–4.
80. Vahlquist A, Peterson PA, Wibell L, Metabolism of the vitamin A transporting protein complex. I. Turnover studies in normal persons and in patients with chronic renal failure. *Eur J Clin Invest* (1973) **3**: 352–62.
81. Grønhøj Larsen F, Nielsen-Kudsk F, Jakobsen P et al, Pharmacokinetics of etretinate in psoriatic patients with liver fibrosis. *Pharmacol Toxicol* (1989) **65**: 393–7.
82. Grønhøj Larsen F, Pharmacokinetics of etretinate and acitretin with special reference to treatment of psoriasis. *Acta Derm Venereol (Stockh)* (1994) **74** (suppl 190) 1–33.
83. Ellis CN, Kang S, Vinik AI et al, Glucose and insulin responses are improved in patients with psoriasis during therapy with etretinate. *Arch Dermatol* (1987) **123**: 471–5.
84. Hartmann D, Forgo I, Duback UG et al, Effect of acitretin on the response to an intravenous glucose tolerance test in healthy volunteers (1992) **42**: 523–8.
85. Garbe C, Hyperkeratotische Form des Morbus Darier und Epilepsie, Weitgehende Risistenz auf synthetische Retinoide. *Z Hautkr* (1984) **59**: 1263–4.
86. Mohammed KN, Unresponsiveness to etretinate during anticonvulsant therapy. *Dermatology* (1992) **185**: 79.
87. Zachariae H, Dangers of methotrexate/etretinate combination therapy (letter). *Lancet* (1988) **i**: 422.
88. Harrison PV, Peat M, James R et al, Methotrexate and retinoids in combination for psoriasis. *Lancet* (1987) **ii**: 512.
89. Larsen FG, Nielsen-Kudsk F, Jakobsen P et al, Interaction of etretinate with methotrexate pharmacokinetics in psoriatic patients. *J Clin Pharmacol* (1990) **30**: 802–7.

90. Shuttleworth D, Marks R, Griffin PJA et al, Treatment of cutaneous neoplasia with etretinate in renal transplant recipients. *Q J Med* (1988) **257**: 717–25.
91. Ali Shah I, Whiting PH, Omar G et al, The effects of retinoids and terbinafine on the human hepatic microsomal metabolism of cyclosporin. *Br J Dermatol* (1993) **129**: 395–8.
92. Webber IR, Back DJ, Effect of etretinate on cyclosporin metabolism in vitro. *Br J Dermatol* (1993) **128**: 42–4.
93. Vahlquist C, Olsson AG, Lindholm A, Vahlquist A, Effects of gemfibrozil (Lopid) on hyperlipidemia in acitretin treated patients: Results of a double-blind cross-over study. *Acta Derm Venereol* (1995) **75**: 377–80.
94. Osterle LS, Langtry JAA, Jones S et al, Reduced therapeutic effect of warfarin caused by etretinate. *Br J Dermatol* (1991) **124**: 505.
95. Hartmann D, Mosberg H, Weber W, Lack of effect of acitretin on the hypothrombinemic action of phenprocoumon in healthy volunteers. *Dermatologica* (1989) **178**: 33–6.
96. Bun H, Berbis P, Durand A et al, Plasma kinetics of acitretin in combination with 8-methoxy psoralen and UVA therapy in psoriatic patients. In: *FIP 89, 49th International Congress of Pharmaceutical Sciences of FIP*, 4–9 Sept, 1989, Munich, Germany, p 214.
97. Beani JC, Bonnot D, Berthod F et al, Influence des rètinoides sur la biodisponibilité du methoxy-8-psoralene. *Ann Dermatol Venereol* (1991) **118**: 273–5.
98. Muindi JRF, Frankel SR, Huselton C, DeGrazia F, Garland WA, Warrell RP Jr, Clinical pharmacology of oral all-*trans*-retinoic acid in patients with acute promyelocytic leukemia. *Cancer Res* (1992) **52**: 2138–42.
99. Muindi JRF, Young CW, Warrell RP Jr, Clinical pharmacology of all *trans* retinoic acid. *Leukemia* (1994) **8** (suppl 3): 516–21.
100. Adamson PC, Bailey J, Pluda J et al, Pharmacokinetics of all-*trans*-retinoic acid administered on an intermittent schedule. *J Clin Oncol* (1995) **13**: 1238–41.
101. Ott F, Bollag W, Geiger JM, Efficacy of low-dose tretinoin (all-*trans*-retinoic acid) in lichen planus. *Dermatology* (1996) **192**: 334–6.
102. Loewen GR, Warrell RP Jr, Hawkins MJ et al, Pharmacokinetics of LGD1057 (9-*cis*-retinoic acid) in patients with cancer. *Pharm Res* (1995) **12** (9, suppl S-102) meeting report.
103. Sass JO, Masgrau E, Saurat JH, Nau H, Metabolism of oral 9-*cis*-retinoic acid in the Human. *Drug Metab Dispos* (1995) **23**: 887–91.

5 Psoriasis: systemic retinoid treatment

Nicholas J Lowe

Introduction

Systemic retinoids are an important form of therapy for patients with more severe and recalcitrant types of psoriasis. The retinoids are usually best prescribed with adjunctive therapy, such as ultraviolet therapy, which often reduces the dosage and duration of retinoid therapy.

Pustular psoriasis

Several studies have confirmed the efficacy of etretinate treatment for different types of severe psoriasis.[1–11] Pustular forms of psoriasis are more responsive to systemic retinoid monotherapy than chronic plaque and erythrodermic psoriasis which respond more slowly.[12] With plaque and erythrodermic psoriasis it is possible to enhance the response to therapy by combining retinoids with other treatments.

When etretinate is used as monotherapy for generalized pustular psoriasis the initial dose required is 1 mg/kg per day. A rapid resolution of generalized pustular psoriasis is achieved usually within 10 days of initiating etretinate which is probably the drug of first choice for the treatment of this condition (Figure 5.1). One advantage with etretinate for this condition over methotrexate is the absence of acute effects on the peripheral blood count. Methotrexate can occasionally produce leukopenia in patients with generalized pustular psoriasis and this can lead to a major toxicity risk in these patients. After the clearance of pustulation with a retinoid, the psoriasis can continue to be controlled with a gradual reduction in etretinate dose,[13] but some patients will relapse, developing plaque psoriasis. In these patients, alternative forms of treatment, for example, ultraviolet or PUVA therapy, can be instituted in combination with etretinate gradually to reduce the dose of etretinate or acitretin. In fertile women, etretinate should be avoided even for generalized pustular psoriasis. In such cases oral isotretinoin at doses of about 1.5 mg/kg per day may be used as an alternative to etretinate to control the pustulation. Isotretinoin is generally much less effective than etretinate in the treatment of exfoliative or plaque psoriasis, and in fertile women with these types of psoriasis it is sometimes justifiable to combine isotretinoin with

Part of this chapter is adapted with permission from Lowe NJ, *Practical psoraisis therapy*, 2nd edn. Mosby Yearbook: St Louis, 1992.

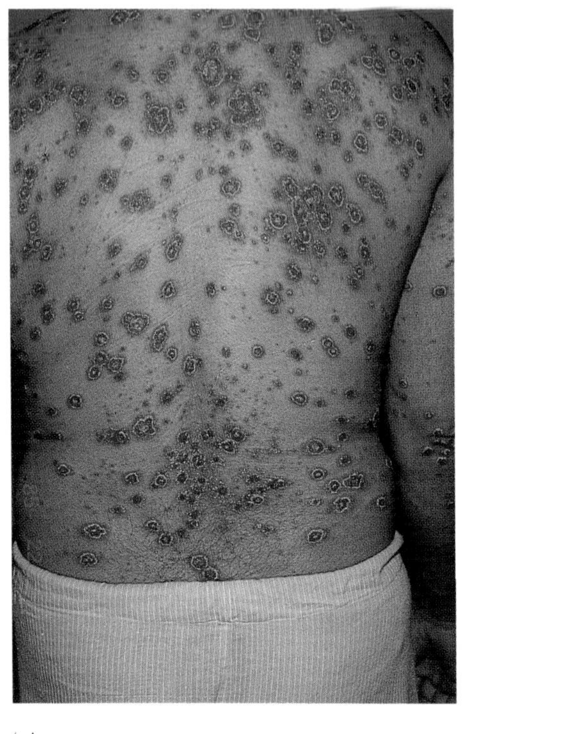

(a)

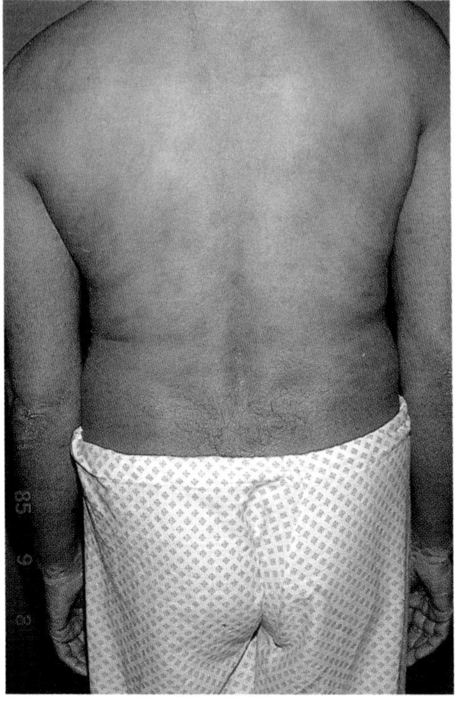

(b)

Figure 5.1

Patient with generalized pustular psoriasis **(a)** before and **(b)** after treatment with etretinate 1 mg/kg per day for 10 days.

other forms of treatment such as topical corticosteroid (for exfoliative psoriasis) or ultraviolet or PUVA phototherapy (for plaque psoriasis) to achieve more rapid control and greater psoriasis clearance. Acitretin is more rapidly excreted and is as effective as etretinate but, as described later in this chapter, in a proportion of patients, some of the acitretin is esterified to etretinate.

Another situation in which both etretinate and isotretinoin are effective in combination with PUVA phototherapy is palmoplantar pustular psoriasis, particularly where there is significant hyperkeratosis or severe pustulation. Retinoid therapy reduces the degree of hyperkeratosis and pustulation. It is also an effective adjunct to ultraviolet therapy.

Exfoliative psoriasis

In exfoliative erythrodermic psoriasis, etretinate or acitretin are also used at a dose of approximately 1 mg/kg per day. It is an advantage to use emollients frequently and topical

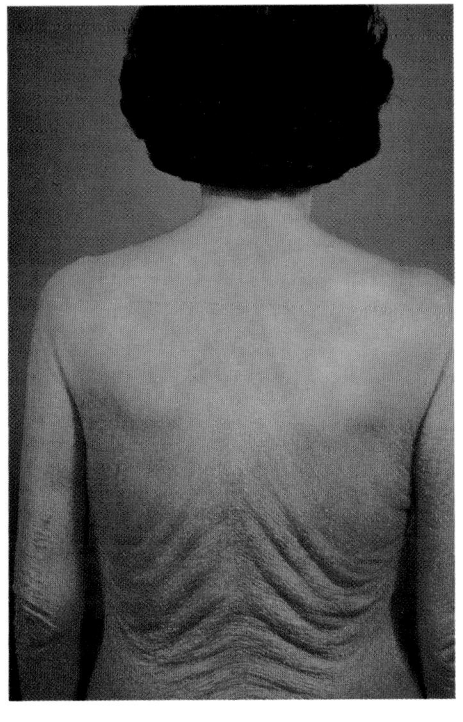

(a)

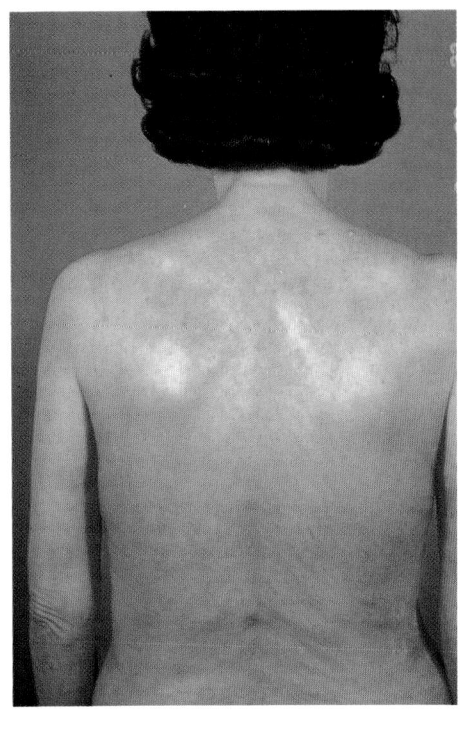

(b)

Figure 5.2

Patient with exfoliative psoriasis **(a)** before and **(b)** after treatment with etretinate.

corticosteroids, for example, triamcinolone acetonide (0.025–0.5% cream or ointment) under an occlusive suit, to achieve more rapid resolution of psoriasis.

Rarely, patients with severe exfoliative erythrodermic psoriasis may need to use a combination of etretinate with methotrexate. This combination should only rarely be used and, when it is, only with careful monitoring.

Another option for the treatment of exfoliative psoriasis is to use methotrexate or cyclosporin therapy to achieve a rapid improvement after which the methotrexate or cyclosporin is reduced and low doses of etretinate (0.25–0.5 mg/kg per day) or acitretin (0.25–0.5 mg/kg) introduced (Figure 5.2).

Combination therapy for moderate to severe plaque psoriasis

In patients with severe plaque psoriasis, particularly if the condition is extensive with hyperkeratosis, the use of a retinoid plus other forms of treatment, particularly

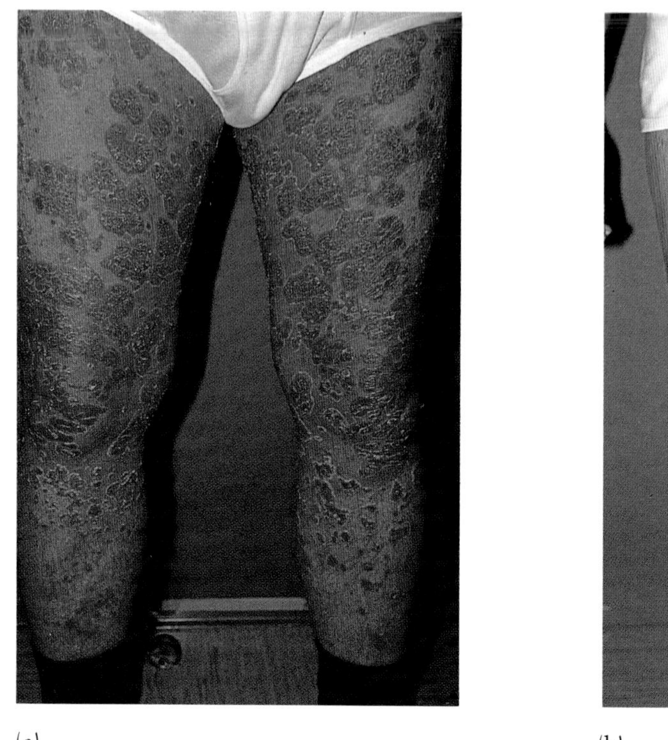

(a)

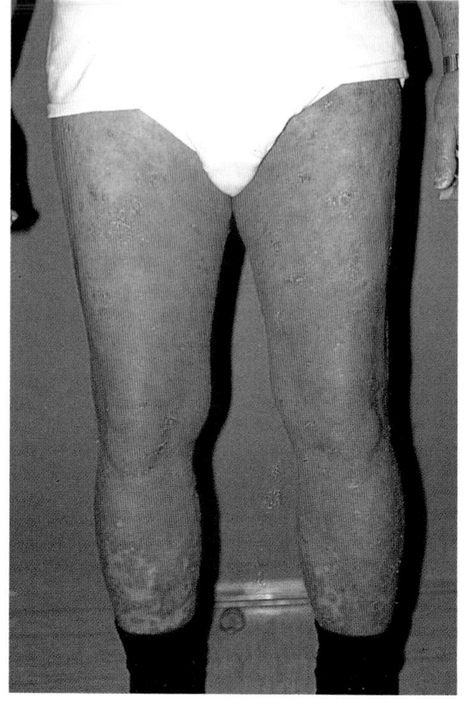

(b)

Figure 5.3

Patient with severe psoriasis **(a)** before and **(b)** after treatment with etretinate.

phototherapy, has been shown to be highly effective. The dose of retinoid or amount of alternative therapy required when used separately can be reduced if used in combination. A response to the etretinate/topical corticosteroid combination is shown in Figure 5.3.

Etretinate or acitretin and ultraviolet or PUVA phototherapy

For combination therapy the optimum doses are etretinate 0.5 mg/kg per day or acitretin 0.3 mg/kg per day, either 2 weeks prior to starting phototherapy or at the same time. The increases in ultraviolet radiation should be more gradual and cautious than in patients not taking systemic retinoid because of an increased risk of ultraviolet radiation-induced erythema. This is not a true photosensitivity, but probably represents increased epidermal transmission of the ultraviolet radiation because of altered optical properties of the stratum corneum caused by the retinoid (Figures 5.4 and 5.5).

The use of PUVA with etretinate has been studied by several investigators.[14–17] The majority of patients receiving the combination improve more quickly than with PUVA

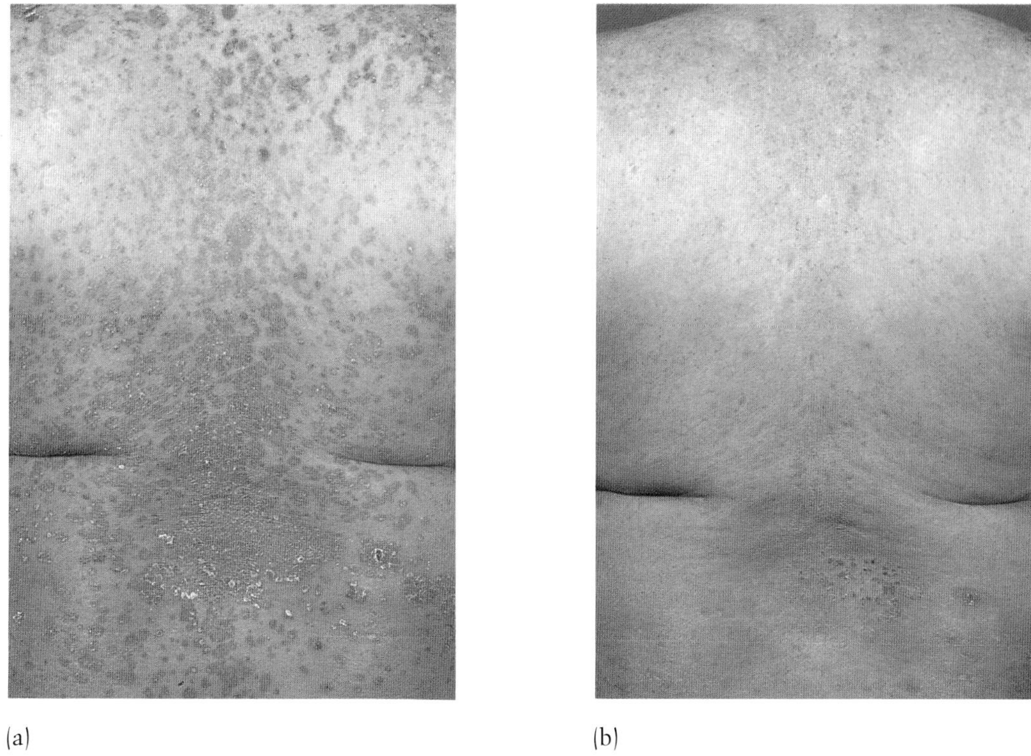

Figure 5.4

Patient with psoriasis **(a)** before and **(b)** after treatment with etretinate plus UVB.

alone or etretinate alone. In addition, the total number of ultraviolet radiation exposures can be reduced. Following clearance of psoriasis various maintenance regimens have been employed. Etretinate administered in low maintenance doses can be effective, or etretinate therapy can be stopped and maintenance therapy undertaken solely with PUVA.

Lauharanta et al[14] investigated the use of the combination of etretinate and PUVA in 80 patients with psoriasis and showed a significantly greater improvement with the combination compared with each therapy alone. Side-effects seen in the patients treated with etretinate consisted mostly of dryness of the lips and mucous membranes. Doses of UVA were significantly reduced as compared with PUVA treatment and maximal efficacy with PUVA was achieved if etretinate was initiated at least 3 weeks beforehand.

Grupper and Beretti[15] evaluated the effects of various etretinate/PUVA combinations as well as etretinate alone. A total of 126 patients with psoriatic lesions covering an average of 60 per cent of the whole body were treated. The majority of the cases treated (84 per cent) were psoriasis vulgaris (plaque type). Others were guttate (8 per cent), erythrodermic (9 per cent) and pustular (1 per cent) types of psoriasis. Patients were treated according

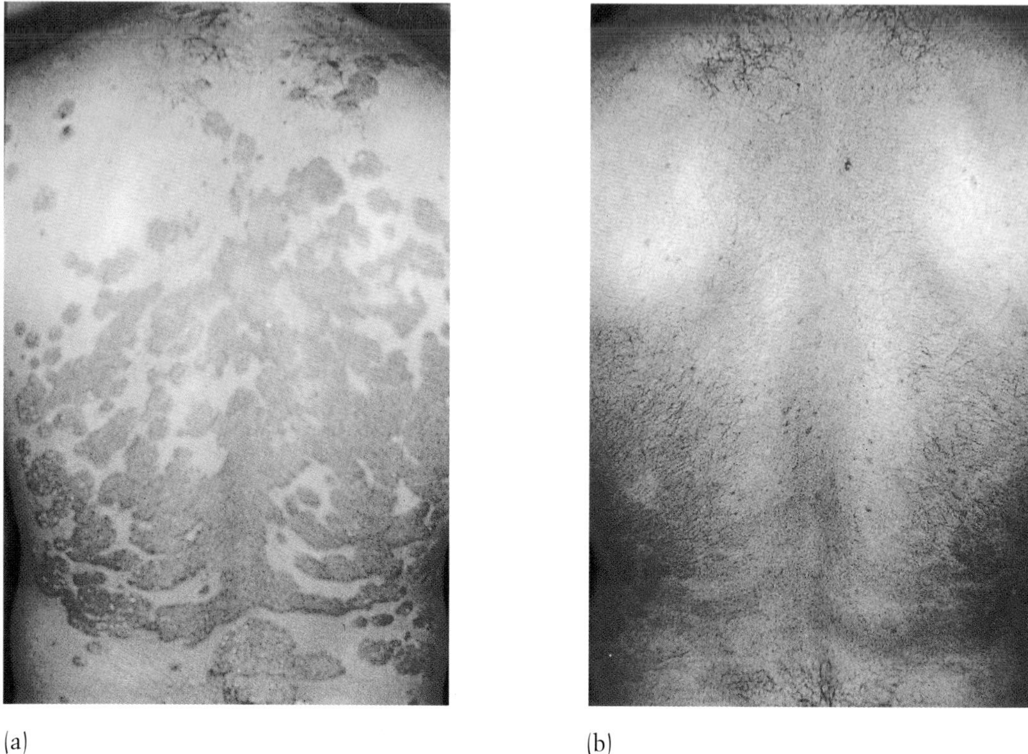

(a) (b)

Figure 5.5

Patient with chronic severe plaque psoriasis **(a)** before and **(b)** 4 weeks after acitretin plus suberythogenic UVB.

to five different protocols, three of them combining etretinate with PUVA. The most effective results were obtained with the following combination schedule. Etretinate alone was administered at a dose of 1 mg/kg per day for 2 weeks. On the 15th day, standard PUVA therapy was begun while the etretinate dose was reduced progressively to 0.75, 0.50 or 0.25 mg/kg per day. PUVA therapy was reduced to a standard maintenance schedule and etretinate withdrawn. This combination therapy made recovery possible for over 70 per cent of the complete or relative failures of PUVA therapy.

Reasons for combining PUVA and systemic retinoids therefore include:

(1) less time needed to achieve clearing;
(2) the number of treatments and duration of PUVA therapy may be reduced;
(3) the possibility of reduction or cessation of etretinate therapy before the occurrence of side-effects such as alopecia or hyperlipidaemia.

Isotretinoin plus UVB or PUVA therapy may be considered for use in fertile women with recalcitrant plaque psoriasis. Acitretin and ultraviolet[18] or PUVA phototherapy has

Table 5.1 **Dosing outline for systemic retinoids in psoriasis**

Indication	*Retinoid*	*Initial dose range (mg/kg per day)*	*Chronic dose (mg/kg per day)*
Generalized pustular psoriasis	Etretinate*	0.75–1.0	0.25–0.5
	Isotretinoin**	1.0–2.0	Not indicated
	Acitretin***	0.5–0.75	0.125–0.25
Exfoliative psoriasis	Etretinate*	0.75–1.0	0.25–0.5
	Isotretinoin**	1.0–1.5	Not indicated
	Acitretin***	0.5–0.75	0.125–0.25
Plaque psoriasis (combination therapy)	Etretinate*	0.5–0.75	0.25–0.5
	Isotretinoin**	1.0–1.5	Not indicated
	Acitretin***	0.25–0.5	0.125–0.25

*Not in fertile women.
**Fertile women in the USA as of 1993.
***Pending approval by the US Food and Drug Administration.

been shown to be superior to either alone. Patients clear more completely with fewer treatments and at a lower acitretin dose. The optimum dose of acitretin is usually 0.25 mg/kg per day, either prior to or at the start of ultraviolet phototherapy. Again, a more cautious increase in ultraviolet and PUVA dosing is required to avoid unwanted radiation-induced erythema, as with etretinate/phototherapy combinations. Acitretin is discussed more completely later in this chapter. See Table 5.1 for suggested oral dosages.

Other systemic retinoids

Arotinoid ethyl ester

Among the newer retinoids currently being evaluated for psoriasis and other diseases are the arotinoid esters. For example, various studies in Europe have shown arotinoid ethyl ester to be potent in very low doses in psoriasis and psoriatic arthritis. In general, it appears to have similar side-effects to etretinate with the possible exception of a reduced risk of hyperlipidaemia. Long-term studies have not been reported with this drug so it is not yet known whether its side-effect profile under chronic usage is different from that of etretinate.

Acitretin

Acitretin (Ro-10-1670) was previously known as etretin. It is an acid metabolite of etretinate. This drug has been evaluated in the USA and Europe and has been shown to be effective in psoriasis.[19] Acitretin was developed because it was thought to be cleared from the body more

Table 5.2 Pharmacokinetics of etretinate and acitretin

Bioavailability	Acitretin Etretinate	36–95% 36–70%
Protein binding	Acitretin – albumin Etretinate – lipoproteins	
Lipid binding	Etretinate 50 times greater than acitretin	
Elimination rate	Acitretin cleared 50 times faster than etretinate*	

*Metabolized partly to etretinate if taken with alcohol.

rapidly than etretinate as it is not lipid bound. One reason to desire rapid clearance of these drugs is because of the risk of teratogenicity. Etretinate should not be used in women of childbearing years because of its persistence in the lipid stores in the body after discontinuation of therapy; this could lead to fetal damage, even if conception occurred several months to years after discontinuation. It was hoped that acitretin, because of its rapid clearance, might be an appropriate form of treatment for women of childbearing potential provided that contraceptive precautions were taken during the course of therapy and probably for 2 months after discontinuation. The drug is currently available in several countries, but in the USA as of September 1996 FDA approval of this agent was delayed because of the possible presence of

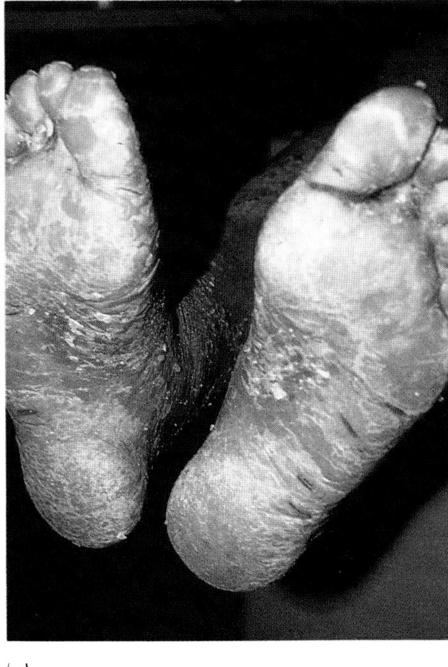

(a)

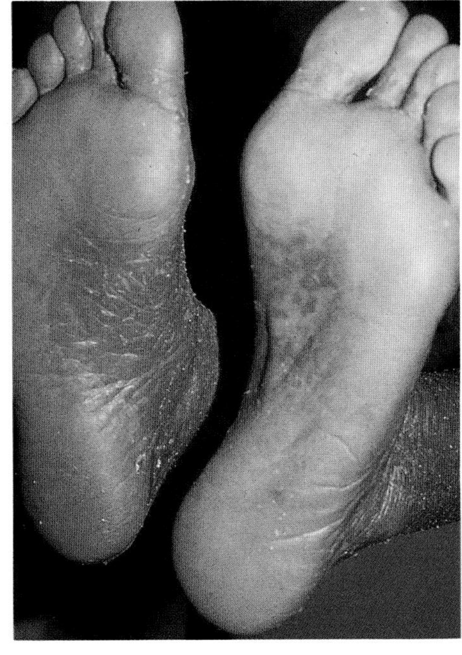

(b)

Figure 5.6

Patient with AIDS and severe psoriasis of feet **(a)** before and **(b)** after treatment with acitretin.

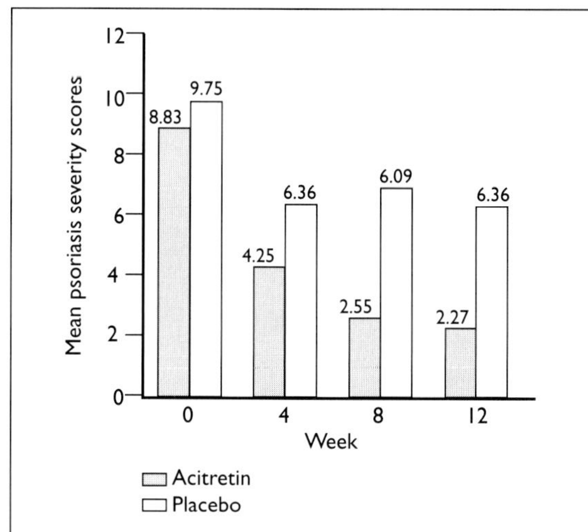

Figure 5.7

Histogram showing the mean psoriasis severity scores in a study of suberythogenic UVB and either acitretin or placebo oral therapy showing the benefits of acitretin UVB combination. Severity psoriasis score: 0, none; 1, mild; 2, moderate; 3, severe; 4, very severe. Potential additive total score = 12

etretinate-like metabolites being found in studies in Europe. There may be several reasons for the occurrence of those metabolites including the possibility that acitretin is esterified to etretinate in the presence of alcohol. Further studies are progressing to explore this problem (Table 5.2).

The toxicity profile of acitretin mimics that of etretinate. Effective drug doses are somewhat lower than etretinate. In various studies the optimum dose of acitretin as monotherapy has been shown to be approximately 0.5–0.6 mg/kg per day (Figure 5.6). When it is used as monotherapy, it is highly effective in generalized pustular psoriasis. As with etretinate in patients with severe plaque psoriasis and exfoliative psoriasis, it is ideally used in combination with other forms of therapy at doses of 0.25–0.5 mg/kg per day (Figure 5.7). Recent studies have confirmed the value of combining acitretin and UVB.[18] Other possible therapies to combine with acitretin include topical therapy and PUVA.

Toxicity of systemic retinoids

Mucocutaneous toxicity

Mucocutaneous toxicity occurs with all of the systemic retinoids.[20] The common mucocutaneous side-effects in order of frequency are mucosal dryness, skin peeling, diffuse alopecia, nail drystrophy, stickiness of the skin, loss of body hair and a change in skin colour. Patients frequently find these extremely difficult to accept. Rapid reduction in retinoid therapy is desirable to reduce the impact on patients of these toxicity problems (Table 5.3; Figures 5.8–5.10).

Table 5.3 **Percentage of patients with side-effects to etretinate**

Signs and symptoms	*Percentage of patients*
Chapped lips	100
Dry nasal mucus	100
Hair loss	30
Dry skin	100
Skin fragility	40
Palm/sole peeling	60
Bruising	20
Fingertip peeling	75
Thirst	30
Nosebleed	10
Sticky/clammy skin	20
Bone/joint pain	5
Irritation of eyes	15
No change	20

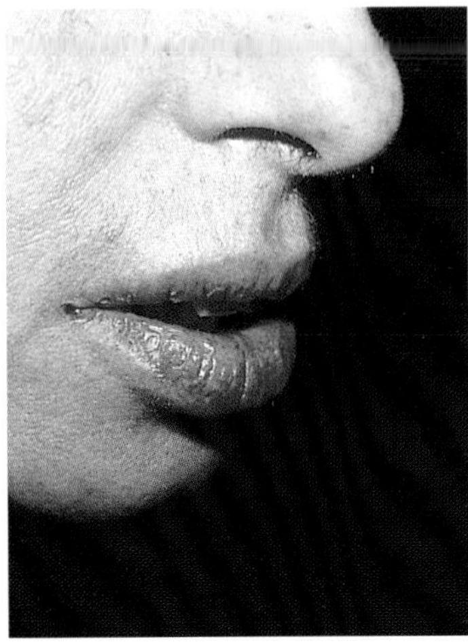

Figure 5.8

Retinoid cheilitis in a patient taking etretinate.

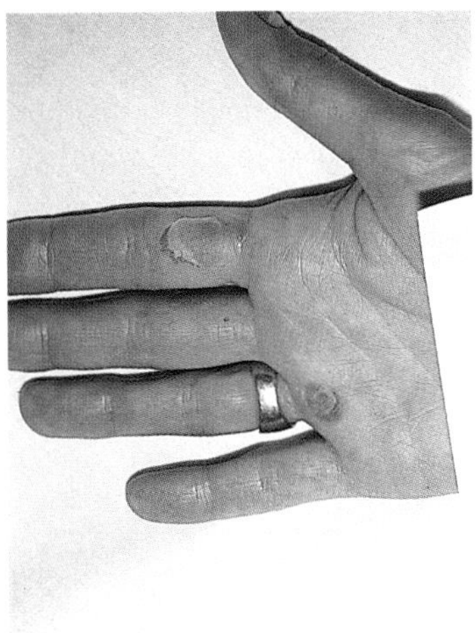

Figure 5.9

Skin fragility erosions in a patient taking etretinate.

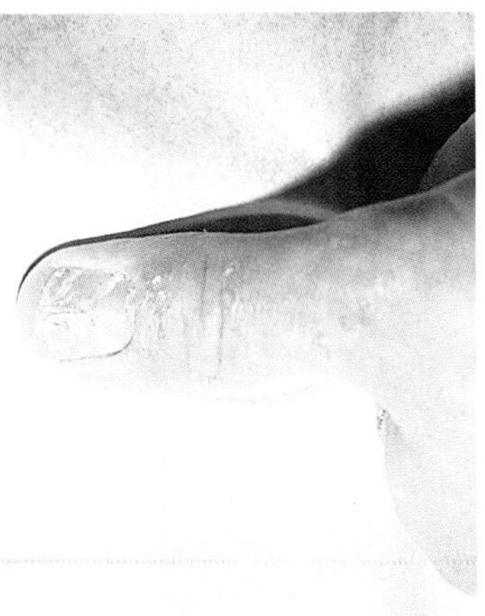

Figure 5.10

Etretinate-induced median nail dystrophy.

Hyperlipidaemia

Hyperlipiademia occurs in approximately 25 per cent of patients. This is occasionally severe with triglyceride values reaching five to eight times normal, but usually the values are two to three times normal. There are a variety of ways to manage this hyperlipidaemia including low-fat diets, reduced alcohol intake and the use of polyunsaturated fish-oil supplements. Should the hyperlipidaemia remain, then a cessation of retinoid therapy or a reduction in dose may be required.

Some patients develop muscle pain and myalgia with or without an elevation of creatine phosphokinase. In general, it is wise for patients to avoid excessive muscle exercise, particularly weight lifting and vigorous aerobic exercise, while on etretinate as this may increase the risk of muscle pain and myalgia.

Ocular toxicity

Ocular toxicity does not appear to be a major problem with acitretin or etretinate, although rare cases of disturbances of colour vision have been recorded. Unpublished observations carried out in two centres in the USA examined the possibility of night blindness in patients on acitretin therapy, but no significant changes were noted.

Skeletal toxicity

There is a concern that long-term high-dose etretinate therapy is associated with skeletal and ligamentous calcification and hyperostosis. There appears to be a cumulative threshold dose of 25–30 g etretinate below which skeletal toxicity is not seen radiographically (Lowe NJ, unpublished data).

It is the author's opinion that patients who are on etretinate (in excess of the threshold dose) should undergo selective radiographic examination to search for hyperostosis. The radiographic views should include those sites most likely to show ligamentous calcification or skeletal hyperostosis, that is, the lateral spine, hips, ankles and knees. Further long-term studies in larger populations are required to determine the relative incidence of skeletal changes during chronic acitretin therapy.

Frequency of follow-up

Blood investigations should include a full blood count, and a complete biochemistry profile including liver enzymes, renal function, triglyceride, cholesterol, high-density lipoprotein and creatine phosphokinase.[21] These investigations should be repeated initially every 2 weeks while on clearance dosages, reducing to monthly or 2-monthly assessments depending on the maintenance dose required. There is presently no requirement for liver biospy (Table 5.4).

Guidelines for the use of systemic retinoids in psoriasis

1. Etretinate can be prescribed for male patients or postmenopausal female patients. Premenopausal fertile women should not be treated with etretinate but can be considered for acitretin or isotretinoin therapy providing they use adequate contraception during therapy and for 1 month (for isotretinoin) or 24 months (for acitretin) after discontinuation.

Table 5.4 Suggested tests for systemic retinoid patients

Pre-treatment tests	
Blood/CBC	Triglyceride*
Liver function	Cholesterol*
Treatment tests	
Repeat every 2 weeks during first 6 weeks' clearing doses (see Table 5.2)	
Repeat every 8 weeks when on low-dose maintenance dosages (see Table 5.1)	
Skeletal radiographs	
To exclude hyperostosis if patient needs continued etretinate after 12 months; then after 25 g of etretinate repeat every year during maintenance etretinate	
Pregnancy tests	
Fertile female patients treated with isotretinoin or acitretin (if available) will need pre-treatment pregnancy test and repeated pregnancy test every month of therapy	

*12-hour fasting blood.

2. Careful pre-treatment and screening should be carried out to exclude the possibility of hyperlipidaemia. Previous adverse reaction to etretinate should be considered as a possible contraindication to the use of acitretin. However, if the patient's condition warrants the use of acitretin, a cautious therapeutic trial would be justified.
3. Retinoids should be considered as monotherapy in generalized pustular psoriasis.
4. Combination therapy of etretinate, acitretin (or isotretinoin) with UVB or PUVA phototherapy is advised in severe plaque psoriasis and localized recalcitrant palmoplantar psoriasis, including local pustular psoriasis of the palms and soles.

Topical retinoids in psoriasis

Topical retinoids have been shown to be highly effective in a number of different skin diseases, including acne and disorders of keratinization such an ichthyoses, as well as in the treatment of photoaged skin. A review of the literature reveals that topical tretinoin has also been shown to be effective in psoriasis. The main disadvantage of retinoic acid therapy in psoriasis is skin irritation. As a result, it has largely been abandoned and a search for retinoid analogues has resulted in agents that retain a retinoid-like effect with less skin irritation. Recent studies with a topical acetylenic retinoid have shown this agent to be effective in psoriasis, and it is hoped that the effectiveness of this or similar agents in the treatment of psoriasis will be confirmed when used either as monotheraphy or in combination with phototherapy.

The acetylenic retinoid has been named tazarotene. Further studies in 1995 and 1996 confirmed this to be effective for psoriasis, and this is discussed further in Chapter 6. Further research into use of tazarotene plus phototherapy and other combinations of therapy are indicated.

References

1. Dahl B, Mollenbach K, Reymann F, Treatment of psoriasis vulgaris with a new retinoic acid derivative RO-10-9359. *Dermatologica* (1977) **154**: 261–7.
2. Frederiksson T, Pettersson U, Severe psoriasis oral therapy with a new retinoid. *Dermatologica* (1970) **157**: 238–44.
3. Fritsch P, Oral retinoids in dermatology. *Int J Dermatol* (1981) **20**: 314–29.

4. Fritsch P, Rauschmeier W, Zussner C, Arotinoid in the treatment of psoriatic arthropathy. *Dermatologica* (1984) **169**(4): 250 (abstract).
5. Glazer S, Roenigk HH, RO-10-8359 in psoriasis. Study of effectiveness and potential hepatoxicity. *J Invest Dermatol* (1981) **76**: 303.
6. Kaplan RP, Russel DH, Lowe NJ, Etretinate therapy for psoriasis. *J Am Acad Dermatol* (1983) **8**: 95–102.
7. Keddie F, Use of vitamin A in the treatment of cutaneous disease. *Arch Dermatol Syphilol* (1983) **58**: 64–102.
8. Lowe NJ, Kaplan R, Breeding J, Etretinate treatment of psoriasis inhibits epidermal ornithine decarboxylate. *J Am Acad Dermatol* (1982) **6**: 697–8.
9. Orfanos C, Oral retinoids: present status. *Br J Dermatol* (1980) **103**: 473–82.
10. Rosenthal M, Retinoids in der behandlung von psoriasis-arthritis. *Schweiz Med Wochenschr* (1979) **109**: 1912–14.
11. Sofen H, Moy R, Lowe NJ, Isotretinoin for generalized pustular psoriasis. *Lancet* (1984) **i**: 40.
12. Voorhees JJ, Orfanos EE, Oral retinoids. *Arch Dermatol* (1981) **117**: 418–21.
13. Dubertret L, Chastang C, Beylot C et al, Maintenance treatment of psoriasis by Tigason: a double-blind randomized clinical trial. *Br J Dermatol* (1985) **113**: 323–30.
14. Lauharanta J, Geiger JM, Aromatic retinoid (RO-10-9359), re PUVA in PUVA in the treatment of psoriasis. In: Orafanos CE, Braun-Falco O, Faber EM et al (eds). *Retinoids: advances in basic research and therapy.* Springer: Berlin, 1981, pp 201–3.
15. Grupper C, Berretti B, Treatment of psoriasis by oral PUVA therapy combined with aromatic retinoid (RO 10-9359; Tigaon®). *Dermatologica* (1981) **162**: 404–13.
16. Michaelsson G, Noren P, Vahlquist A, Combined therapy with oral retinoid and PUVA baths in severe psoriasis. *Br J Dermatol* (1978) **99**: 221-2.
17. Clark T, Combined etretinate and PUVA to reduce UVA dose side effects. *Dermatol Times* (1987) **8**(5): 30,32.
18. Lowe NJ, Prystowsky J, Armstrong R, Acitretin plus UVB therapy for psoriasis. *J Am Acad Dermatol* (1991) **4**: 591-4.
19. Kingston T, Matt L, Lowe NJ, Etretin therapy for severe psoriasis. *Arch Dermatol* (1987) **123**: 55–8.
20. David M, Lowe NJ, New retinoids for dermatologic diseases, uses and toxicity. *Dermatol Clin* (1988) **6**: 539–52.
21. Lew-Kaya DA, Kruegger GG, Lowe NJ et al, Safety and efficacy of a new retinoid gel in the treatment of psoriasis. *J Invest Dermatol* (1992) **98**: 600 (abstract).

6 Topical retinoids for psoriasis

Ronald Marks and Nicholas Lowe

Introduction

The retinoids possess a remarkable range of activities and clinical uses. One or another of these analogues of vitamin A (retinol) has been shown to be effective in treating disorders of acne, psoriasis, skin cancer, chronic photodamage and keratinization. How their therapeutic actions are accomplished is not always clear, although it seems that the retinoid agent binds to nuclear receptors in the 'target tissues' as an essential first step. After binding, gene expression is modulated so that rogue disordered tissues are persuaded to differentiate along more orderly and normal pathways. This may not be the whole story as it is believed that in some situations non-receptor-mediated effects do occur.

Whatever the details of the mode of action of the retinoids in the different disorders for which they are prescribed, these potent molecules would be even more useful if their pharmacological effects were not accompanied by undesirable, toxic side-effects. This realization has prompted retinoid chemists, and the pharmaceutical companies for whom they work, to synthesize new retinoid molecules with greater sensitivity for particular retinoid receptor profiles (different tissues have different receptor profiles). It is reasoned that it is more likely that there will be greater effects on target tissues with the matching set of receptor sites, and consequently there will be less potential for adverse side-effects.

New retinoids that can be used topically seem likely to have special appeal as there should be even less opportunity for causing systemic intoxication and thus greatly reduce the likelihood of teratogenicity, which is always a danger with retinoid therapy. Topical treatments are needed for the large majority of patients with psoriasis, and it is gratifying that there is now one topical retinoid whose therapeutic activity in psoriasis is incontestable. This retinoid will become available in many countries during 1997.

Rationale

The ability of tretinoin to alter abnormal keratinization and to improve scaling skin disorders led Frost and Weinstein[1] to use topical tretinoin for plaque-type psoriasis. They noted a marked improvement in tretinoin-treated sites compared with the placebo-treated areas. Others[2,3,4] also noted that topical tretinoin had a therapeutic effect in psoriasis, but although of interest at that time the irritation caused by the tretinoin inhibited further pharmaceutical development. Topical isotretinoin was found marginally helpful in a study by Bischoff et al,[5] although in one recent unpublished randomized double-blind, placebo-controlled study conducted in Cardiff, Wales, topical isotretinoin applied over 4 weeks only showed a trend to improvement compared with the placebo control without statistical significance (Marks R, Turner R, unpublished data). Meanwhile oral retinoids were developed and were found to be extremely helpful for patients with severe generalized psoriasis so that the interest in the potential of a topical retinoid for limited disease was kept alive. When new retinoid molecules were synthesized and found to be active in animal and in vitro model systems, as well as having acceptable toxicity profiles and activity after topical application, they were submitted to clinical studies in patients with psoriasis very early on. This occurred with a new retinoid molecule synthesized by Allergan Skin Care and given the code name AGN 190168, and later known as tazarotene. In a 14-day study performed by Esgleyes-Ribot et al[6] a 0.05% gel preparation administered twice daily drastically altered the abnormal keratinization in plaque psoriasis. A total of 13 lesions was evaluated both clinically and histochemically in seven patients. There was statistically significant improvement in the clinical signs, even though the treatment period was for only 14 days. Of great interest was the decrease in the abnormal and 'precocious' expression of several markers of epidermal differentiation, including transglutaminase, keratin 16, involucrin and epidermal growth factor receptor. There was also a decrease in the expression of the cellular markers of inflammation, notably intercellular adhesion molecule type I (ICAM-I). These and other studies conducted around this time convinced all concerned that tazarotene would be therapeutically useful in psoriasis.

Chemistry and pharmacology

Figure 6.1 demonstrates the considerable difference in chemical structure of tazarotene compared with retinol. Some authorities have

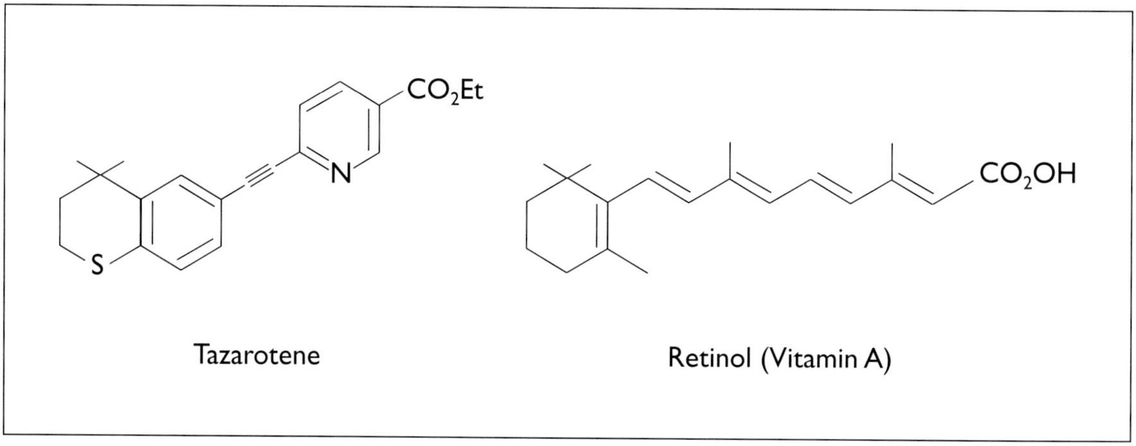

CO_2Et

N

S

Tazarotene

CO_2OH

Retinol (Vitamin A)

Figure 6.1

Chemical structures of tazarotene and retinol.

suggested that, because of the absence of the polyene chain, tazarotene cannot be said to be a true retinoid. In our view this objection is groundless as tazarotene binds avidly to the nuclear retinoic acid receptor, and has all the usual pharmacological actions of retinoid molecules. Figure 6.1 also demonstrates the presence of an unusual feature – the acetylenic bond.

After penetration into the skin, tazarotene is very rapidly transformed to an active metabolite, tazarotenic acid, to the extent that tazarotene should really be regarded as a 'prodrug'. It is excreted in the urine as metabolic oxidative products: the sulfone and sulfoxide.

Safety

There has been an extensive programme of safety testing, and in vitro and in vivo in animals and human volunteer subjects. In addition, therapeutic drug monitoring from clinical trials has greatly extended the information available on the safety of tazarotene.

Animal studies

Single oral doses as large as 2 g/kg caused no adverse effects in rats. Administration for periods of up to 6 months of smaller doses (e.g. 0.25 mg/kg) was well tolerated, but did result in typical retinoid bone toxicity, and in teratogenicity in rats and rabbits. Monkeys also developed bone changes at a dose level of 0.125 mg/kg for a period of 6 months.

Topical application of 0.05% and 0.1% tazarotene gel to multiple species for periods of up to one year did not cause carcinogenic, mutagenic or teratogenic effects. Furthermore, no systemic toxicities resulted from the topical applications in these experiments. The only side-effect was a moderate degree of skin irritation which was predictable as all topical retinoids cause local irritation.

Human studies

Phase I tests on volunteers

Tests assessing the potential of the topical formulations to cause skin irritation, allergic contact sensitization, photoirritancy and photosensitization were conducted in separate panels of normal human volunteer subjects. The cumulative-irritancy test was conducted in 29 subjects by applying the test materials semi-occlusively for 24 hours on 15 occasions over a 21-day period. The test materials included 0.05% and 0.1% tazarotene gels, 0.1% tretinoin cream, 5% benzoyl peroxide gel and 20% azelaic acid cream, and the cumulative irritancy was assessed on a routinely employed arbitrary clinical scoring system.

All the topical retinoids tested caused the same or a similar degree of skin irritation. The potential for allergic contact sensitization was assessed in 181 volunteer subjects using a repeat insult patch test protocol in which nine semi-occlusive applications of 0.05% and 0.1% tazarotene gel were made to the back over a 3-week period. Each patch remained in place for 24 hours. A challenge patch was applied for 24 hours to a previously unexposed area of skin after a 2-week rest period. No instances of sensitization were noted.

The phototoxicity (photoirritancy) and photosensitization potential of 0.05% and 0.1% tazarotene gel were investigated on forearm skin by irradiating one arm with UVA after application of the gels and shielding the other arm from UVR after the tazarotene applications. No photoirritancy or photosensitization was observed.

In summary, the phase I safety tests described above demonstrate that, apart from the expected degree of primary irritation of the same order as seen with all topical retinoids, the topical tazarotene formulations did not seem to have the potential for causing serious skin reactions.

Pharmacokinetics

An important aspect of safety testing is an assessment of the potential that the compound of interest has for penetrating the stratum corneum from the vehicle in which it is formulated and reaching the systemic circulation. In practice the topical preparations are applied to abnormal skin with decreased barrier capacity, but as the state of the barrier is bound to be variable and dependent on site and the stage of disease, and one action of the compound is to improve the barrier anyway, it is more useful to measure the penetration through intact normal skin. Several studies of the percutaneous penetration of tazarotene from 0.05% and 0.1% gels were made. It should be noted that, after topical application, tazarotene undergoes hydrolysis to form its active metabolite tazarotenic acid. Very little parent compound is detected in the plasma. A pivotal investigation was that performed by Franz and colleagues in Arkansas with six normal male volunteer subjects using ^{14}C-labelled tazarotene. The 0.1% gel was applied 'semi-occlusively' at 2 mg/cm^2 to areas of skin on the back, 800 cm^2 in size, and was undisturbed for a 10-hour period. Blood, urine, stool and adhesive tape stratum corneum strip levels of radioactivity were measured at different time points over the next week. The results show that the total amount of radioactivity that penetrated the skin barrier from the topical gel formulation was less than 6 per cent of that applied. It appears that the bulk of this is as the metabolite formed rapidly after penetration into the skin – tazarotenic acid.

In another experiment after a single topical application to 20 per cent of total body surface of 24 healthy subjects, C_{max} and AUC_{0-24h} of tazarotenic acid with 0.1% gel were 40 per cent higher than with 0.5% gel. After 7 days of topical dosing with the 0.1% gel on 20 per cent of total body surface in 24 healthy subjects without occlusion, C_{max} was 0.72 ± 0.58 ng/ml (mean ± SD) occurring 9 hours after the last dose and AUC_{0-24h} was 10.1 ± 7.2 ng h/ml. Systemic absorption was 0.91 ± 0.67 per cent of the applied dose.

In a large pharmacokinetic study simulating typical clinical use for 3 months, daily topical applications of tazarotene gel to lesional skin (mean: 7.2 ± 3.2 to 5.5 ± 4.7% of total body surface area) of 24 psoriatic patients without occlusion yielded C_{max} of 0.45 ± 0.78 ng/ml and AUC_{0-24h} of 5.7 ± 8.5 ng h/ml for the 0.05% gel and C_{max} of 0.83 ± 1.22 ng/ml and AUC_{0-24h} of 11.8 ± 16.0 ng h/ml for the 0.1% gel. Extrapolation of these results to represent dosing on 20 per cent of total body surface area yielded C_{max} of 0.71 ± 0.40 ng/ml and AUC_{0-24h} of 10.2 ± 4.8 ng h/ml for the 0.05% gel, and C_{max} of 2.93 ± 2.89 ng/ml and AUC_{0-24h} of 42.1 ± 37 ng h/ml for the 0.1% gel. Systemic absorption was 1.80 ± 0.81 per cent of the applied dose for the 0.05% gel, and 3.87 ± 3.13 per cent for the 0.1% gel.

During clinical trials for the treatment of psoriasis with the 0.05% and 0.1% gels, plasma tazarotenic acid concentrations from 601 patients ranged from <0.05 ng/ml (below the limit of quantitation) to 6.1 ng/ml. Greater than 90 per cent of these patients with detectable tazarotenic acid had concentrations of less than 1 ng/ml. During clinical trials for the treatment of acne with 0.05% or 0.1% gels, plasma tazarotenic acid concentrations from 92 patients ranged from <0.05 ng/ml to 0.15 ng/ml. Tazarotene and tazarotenic acid are metabolized to sulfoxides, sulfones and other polar metabolites. Both urinary and faecal pathways were found to be equally important for the excretion of tazarotene and metabolites. Tazarotenic acid is highly bound to plasma proteins (>99 per cent).

The large variability in plasma concentrations observed following topical tazarotene application to psoriatic subjects is mainly due to the differences in lesional skin condition and the surface area of application. Both tazarotene and tazarotenic acid undergo rapid systemic elimination, thus limiting the

Table 6.1 Clinical trials evaluating tazarotene in the treatment of psoriasis in the USA

Description	Study design	Duration (weeks)	
		Treatment	Follow-up
Phase II trials (dose-ranging)			
Tazarotene 0.05%, 0.01% gel b.i.d. versus vehicle	R, D-b	6	None
Tazarotene 0.1% or 0.05% gel, daily or b.i.d	R, D-b	8	8
Phase III trials			
Tazarotene 0.1%, 0.05% daily gel versus vehicle	M, R, D-b	12	12
Tazarotene 0.1%, 0.05% gel daily versus flucinonide 0.05% cream b.i.d.	M, R, D-b	12	12

b.i.d., twice daily; D-b, double-blind; M, multicentre; R, randomized.

propensity to distribute to systemic tissues. Since the elimination of half-life is short and intersubject variabilities in apparent clearance and volume of distribution are low, the absorbed drug is eliminated quickly and consistently across the patient population.

In summary it can be said that after topical application only limited amounts are absorbed through the skin (less than 6 per cent). The absorbed compound is rapidly metabolized to the active metabolite, tazarotenic acid, and then excreted. There is no tissue storage component to the pharmacokinetic profile of tazarotene.

Clinical studies of tazarotene

In an extensive series of clinical studies, topically applied tazarotene has been shown to treat mild to moderate plaque psoriasis effectively with acceptable patient tolerability.[6,7,8,9] These studies included two dose-ranging studies, a pivotal vehicle-controlled study, and a comparison with the potent topical corticosteroid, flucinonide (Table 6.1). The authors have been involved in several of these investigations.

Results

Dose-ranging study: tazarotene 0.05% versus 0.01% gel twice daily

Early in development a 0.01% concentration was tested. Tazarotene 0.05% gel had a higher treatment success rate than the vehicle, and was significantly more effective than both the 0.01% gel and vehicle gel in reducing the severity of signs and symptoms. Tazarotene 0.01% gel was the minimal effective dose

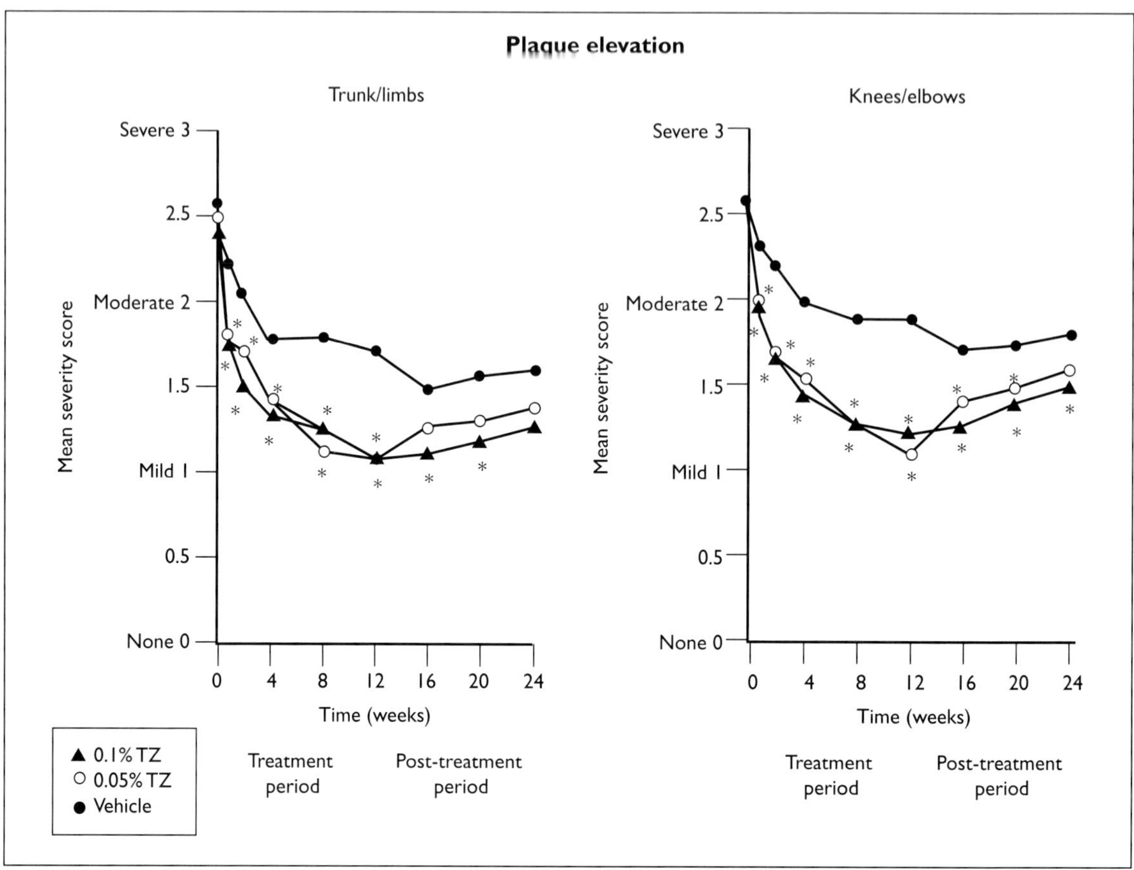

Figure 6.2

Response of patients to different concentrations of tazarotene or vehicle.

and, by the end of the study, the 0.01% gel was more effective than vehicle.[7]

Dose-ranging study: tazarotene 0.05% versus 0.01% gel, once daily versus twice daily

Reductions in the mean severity of signs and symptoms were significant for all four dosage regimens throughout the 8-week treatment period and during the 8-week post-treatment follow-up. Sustained beneficial effects were observed in many patients after treatment was discontinued. Some patients showed continued improvement post-treatment: the number of completely cleared plaques increased from 4 at the end of therapy, to 15 plaques 8 weeks post-treatment.

Pivotal study: tazarotene 0.1% and 0.05% gel versus vehicle, once daily

Tazarotene treated plaques demonstrated clinical improvement as early as one week after the initiation of treatment and was significantly more effective than vehicle in reducing clinical signs of psoriasis during the 12-week treatment period (Figure 6.2). Both tazarotene 0.05% and 0.1% continued to produce improvement during 12 weeks of post-treatment follow-up.

Tazarotene 0.1% and 0.05% gel once daily versus fluocinonide 0.05% cream twice daily

Tazarotene 0.1% gel produced an onset of effect similar to fluocinonide 0.05% cream. After 8 weeks of treatment, no significant differences in lesion severity were observed between tazarotene and fluocinonide for knee and elbow lesions. Compared with twice daily fluocinonide 0.05% cream, once daily tazarotene 0.05% and 0.1% gels were similarly effective in reducing plaque elevation. As expected with a potent corticosteroid, fluocinonide had a significantly greater effect on erythema than tazarotene (Figure 6.3).[2] For lesions overall, treatment success rates were similar but somewhat lower for tazarotene 0.1% than for fluocinonide.

During the post-treatment period, both tazarotene gels demonstrated a more prolonged therapeutic effect than fluocinonide. The cumulative probability of post-treatment relapse was 18 per cent for tazarotene 0.1%, 37 per cent for tazarotene 0.05%, and 55 per cent for fluocinonide ($P<0.05$ versus tazarotene 0.1%).

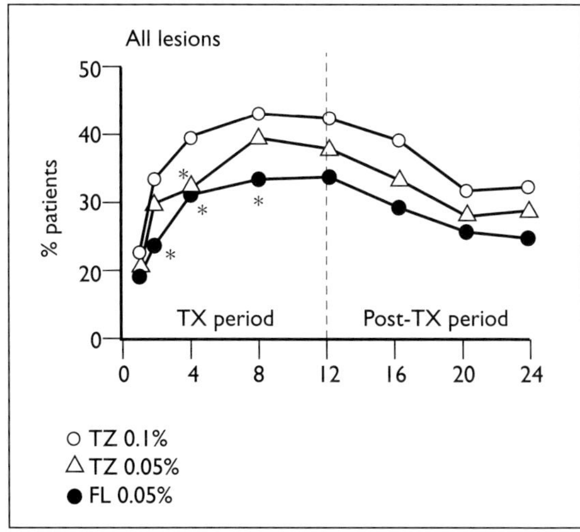

Figure 6.3

Percentage of patients responding to tazarotene or fluocinonide during treatment and post-therapy phase.

Adverse events in clinical use

The only adverse events experienced during the clinical trial programme were the expected irritant reactions observed at the sites of application. In general these reactions were as anticipated with a topical retinoid and were mild and manageable. Local irritation was clearly dose related, especially during the first four weeks of use, and there did appear to be 'accommodation' in that the irritation decreased the longer the tazarotene was used. Itching was the most frequent side-effect, occurring in 20–25 per cent of patients. Burning, erythema and irritation occurred in 10–20 per cent of subjects (Table 6.2). Other unwanted side-effects such as pain, aggravation of the psoriasis, irritant dermatitis and 'desquamation' were noted in 5–10 per cent patients.

There were no serious systemic adverse effects observed in clinical studies involving approximately 2000 patients treated with either the 0.05% gel or the 0.1% gel.

Laboratory safety analyses performed on patients using the 0.1% or 0.05% tazarotene gels for up to one year revealed no clinically significant drug-related changes in standard haematological or biochemical parameters. In view of the bone toxicity associated with oral retinoid drugs, radiological tests were

Table 6.2 Adverse events associated with 0.05% and 0.1% tazarotene gel versus vehicle gel in a phase III study

Adverse event	*Patients*		
	Vehicle	*Tazarotene 0.05%*	*Tazarotene 0.1%*
Itching (%)	8.3	16.7	23.1
Burning (%)	5.6	14.8	18.5
Irritation (%)	0	2.8	9.3
Erythema (%)	0.9	6.5	8.3

performed on 45 patients treated with 0.1% tazarotene gel and 41 patients treated with 0.05% tazarotene gel for periods of up to one year. No significant treatment-related radiological abnormalities were detected. Although reassuring, skeletal abnormalities due to retinoid ingestion generally occur after longer periods (e.g. 2–3 years), and after much higher retinoid exposures.

Despite warnings, three of the female subjects in the clinical trial programme became pregnant while participating in the studies. Two of these subjects were using the tazarotene gel preparations. All three women were delivered of normal healthy children who have subsequently developed normally.

Conclusions

- Tazarotene 0.1% and 0.05% gels applied once daily effectively reduced the severity of psoriatic signs and symptoms.
- Significant clinical improvement was observed as early as 1 week after the beginning of treatment.
- Sustained beneficial effects were observed in some patients for up to 12 weeks after the cessation of therapy.
- Tazarotene was associated with a lower relapse rate compared with fluocinonide after the discontinuation of therapy.

Clinical tips for use of tazarotene gel in psoriasis

This new topical treatment for psoriasis should prove to be a useful addition to our therapeutic armamentarium. Because it has topical retinoid activity and the potential for producing retinoid dermatitis, special care is required for its prescribing and patient instructions to ensure efficacy without skin toxicity.

The ideal patient for tazarotene therapy is the patient with psoriasis plaques on the trunk and limbs (Figure 6.4). Initial treatment should be alternate-day application. If any significant retinoid irritancy is observed, the patient should be advised to delay the next application of the gel for several days and restart application once the irritancy has settled.

Emollient creams should be used frequently between gel applications and may help to prevent the retinoid dermatitis. In patients

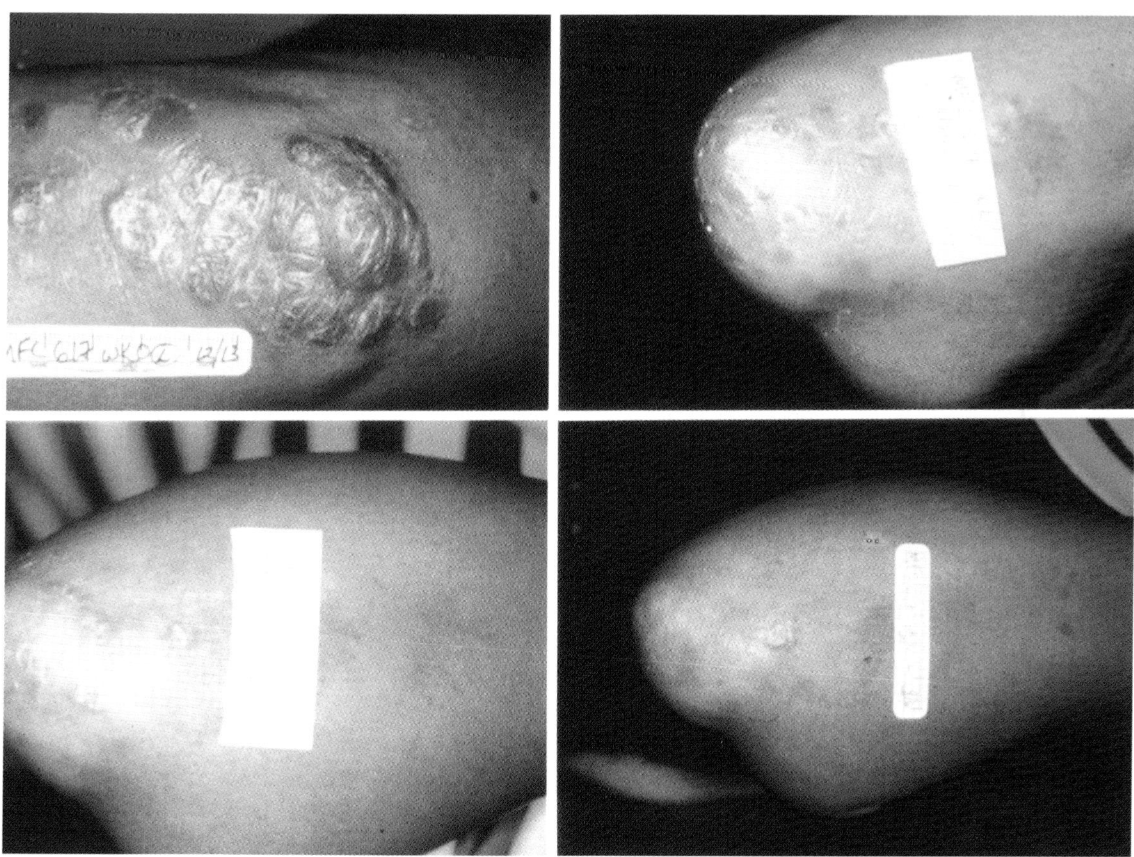

Figure 6.4

Effects of tazarotene gel on plaque psoriasis: (top left) pre-treatment; (top right) after 6 weeks' treatment; (bottom left) after 12 weeks' treatment; (bottom right) 8 weeks post-treatment showing persistent improvement.

who do not experience retinoid dermatitis and in whom psoriasis improvement is slow, tazarotene gel may be applied daily.

Patients who have very inflammatory psoriasis could be initially treated with an ultra potent topical corticosteroid for up to 2 weeks and then tazarotene gel introduced on alternate days. Topical corticosteroids can be used also in patients who develop a painful retinoid dermatitis.

Combination therapy using tazarotene gel plus ultraviolet or PUVA phototherapy is also an alternative to treat patients who have more extensive psoriasis. The tazarotene gel should be applied to the large, more severe psoriasis lesions on alternate days, and the patient should receive ultraviolet therapy at least 3 times weekly or PUVA 2 to 3 times weekly until marginally improved. The use of tazarotene may reduce the amount of UV radiation required to improve the psoriasis. This hypothesis needs to be further explored, but based on experiences with systemic retinoid and ultraviolet combinations[5] it should be effective. Tazarotene gel may also be used as an adjunct for systemic therapy.

Tazarotene gel may be of special value in scalp psoriasis. Here the tazarotene gel is applied overnight and the scalp shampooed in the morning. Alternate nightly application is employed initially. Weekly maintenance scalp therapy with tazarotene gel may be used once maximally improved. Sites that require particular caution when using tazarotene treatment include the skin folds (inguinal and axillary) and the face as these areas may be more likely to develop retinoid dermatitis.

Practical clinical aspects of tazarotene gel

The authors consider tazarotene gel to be a very useful new topical therapy for mild to moderate plaque psoriasis. It is likely to be optimally used by daily or alternate daily application in combination with corticosteroids, moisturisers and other agents such as UVB or PUVA phototherapy. In more severe cases it may be used as a topical adjunctive therapy with systemic treatment. Some patients develop an irritant dermatitis from the gel which can usually be managed by reducing application frequency and alternating with moisturiser or topical corticosteroids.

In summary, tazarotene gel can be used on alternate days initially and if no irritation occurs it can then be applied daily. The use of emollients may reduce irritation. Combinations with topical corticosteroids, phototherapy and systemic therapy may be quite helpful for some patients. Overnight treatments for scalp psoriasis may be useful for stubborn patches.

Summary

There is ample evidence that retinoids have a fundamental effect in psoriasis. They appear to alter the pattern of keratinization and to modulate the expression of markers of the disease. It has long been known that topical tretinoin has some therapeutic activity, but this has not been developed further because of the irritation it produced. In recent years a new acetylenic retinoid has been identified that is active topically. It has been shown that at 0.05% and 0.1% concentrations in a gel formulation tazarotene has excellent therapeutic qualities and has the particular benefit of producing prolonged remission. It has been shown that, although tazarotene possesses the usual toxicity effects of retinoid drugs when administered systemically, it is extremely safe when given topically. Very little is absorbed (less than 6 per cent) and the only adverse side-effects from its use after topical application are the expected degree of skin irritation. Tazarotene may be used as with other retinoids[10] together with phototherapy. This new topical retinoid is likely to be extremely useful in clinical practice for the treatment of plaque-type psoriasis.

References

1. Frost P, Weinstein GD, Topical administration of vitamin A acid for ichthyosiform dermatoses and psoriasis. *J Am Med Assoc* (1969) 207, **10**: 1863–68.
2. Peck GL, Key DJ, Guss SB et al, Topical vitamin A acid in the treatment of psoriasis. *Arch Dermatol* (1973) **107**: 245–8.
3. Günther S, The therapeutic value of retinoic acid in chronic discoid, acute guttate, and erythrodermic psoriasis: clinical observations on twenty-five patients. *Br J Dermatol* (1973) **89**: 515–17.
4. Orfanos CE, Schmidt HW, Mahrle G et al, Retinoic acid in psoriasis: its value for topical therapy with and without corticosteroids. *Br J Dermatol* (1973) **88**: 167–81.
5. Bischoff R, De Jong EMGJ, Rulo HFC et al, Topical application of 13-*cis*-retinoic acid in

the treatment of chronic plaque psoriasis. *Clin Exp Dermatol* (1992) **17**: 9–12.
6. Esgleyes-Ribot T, Chandraratna RA, Lew-Kaya DA et al, Response of psoriasis to a new topical retinoid, AGN 190168. *J Am Acad Dermatol* (1994) **30**: 581–90.
7. Lew-Kaya DA, Kruegger GG, Lowe NJ et al, Safety and efficacy of a new retinoid gel in the treatment of psoriasis (abstract). *J Invest Dermatol* (1992) **98**: 600.
8. Marks R, Early clinical development of tazarotene. *Br J Dermatol* (1996) **135** (suppl 49): 26–31.
9. Weinstein GD, Safety, efficacy and duration of therapeutic effect of tazarotene used in the treatment of plaque psoriasis. *Br J Dermatol* (1996) **135** (suppl 49): 32–6.
10. Lowe NJ, Prystowsky J, Bourget T, Armstrong RB. Acitretin plus UVB therapy for psoriasis. *J Am Acad Dermatol* (1991) **4**: 591–4.

7 Acne and related disorders

Ronald Marks

Introduction

Acne always distresses its victims. It often disables and may even cripple a few patients who have the nodulocystic variety of the disorder. Effective therapies were few and far between before topical all-*trans*-retinoic acid (tretinoin) became available at the beginning of the 1970s. The introduction of this agent and topical isotretinoin more recently has assisted the management of patients with mild to moderate degrees of acne. Of even greater impact has been the development of oral isotretinoin for the treatment of patients with more severe forms of the disease, including the nodulocystic variety. In this chapter I will describe the role of the retinoid drugs in the management of acne as well as problems that may arise in their use and their modes of action. We will also pay some attention to the use of these drugs in the treatment of disorders that traditionally have been described alongside acne, although possibly aetiopathogenetically unrelated, including hidradenitis suppurativa, dissecting folliculitis and rosacea.

Treatment of acne

Use of topical tretinoin

Tretinoin is one of the 'first generation' retinoids and is the carboxylic acid of retinol (vitamin A). It is a natural metabolite and has been in use for the treatment of acne since the beginning of the 1970s but during this time has also been used in the treatment of disorders of keratinization, solar keratoses, non-melanoma skin cancer and even melanoma (see chapters 8 and 9). Topical tretinoin is available as a lotion, cream and gel in concentrations of 0.01%, 0.025%, 0.05% and 0.1%. All concentrations are not available in all the formulations, and in different countries the same range of tretinoin-containing products may not be available. Another preparation has been available since 1995. This is a 0.05% cream formulated to have special emollient properties and for use in photodamage. It should be remembered that tretinoin is a very 'sensitive' molecule and easily broken down by oxidative processes. On no account should the commercially available preparation be diluted or added to, as this will threaten the integrity of the formulation and its therapeutic activity. Oxidation of the tretinoin molecule is aided by high ambient temperatures and by exposure to ultraviolet radiation (UVR). For this reason the preparations should be stored in a cool, sunless place. Storage in a domestic refrigerator at 4°C is ideal. Because of the photodegradation that takes place in sunlight, patients should be instructed not to use a tretinoin preparation if they intend to be exposed outdoors within 1 h of applying it. The breakdown products of tretinoin tend to be yellowish, so that if a preparation has a yellow appearance it should be discarded.

The question is often asked, as it is about most topical agents: how often is it necessary to apply the material to obtain the best results? The empirical and slightly fatuous answer is, at least for topical tretinoin, as often as is necessary in that particular patient. Mostly patients do not need to apply it more than once per day – preferably before going to bed, so that there is no chance of photodegradation. However, there are some patients, particularly fair-complexioned or red-haired individuals, who cannot tolerate daily use (see later) and these might have to use the agent on alternate days.

It is a common mistake to apply anti-acne medications just to the affected area. The whole of the skin of the affected part is probably involved with the acne abnormality – whatever it is – and it seems logical to apply the tretinoin not only to the area with lesions but also to the area of uninvolved skin around the lesions.

Another question that is frequently asked concerns the concurrent use of other medications. There is no objection to prescribing systemic antibiotics at the same time as the topical tretinoin. This is certainly an acceptable practice, and seems entirely appropriate for patients with fairly superficial but inflamed acne lesions affecting more than one site (such as the patient in Figure 7.1). I often recommend the concurrent use of oral tetracycline or erythromycin and topical tretinoin. In such patients it is advisable to start off with the topical tretinoin and then add the oral antibiotics after 4 weeks or so if the therapeutic response has not been as complete as expected. In this way it should be possible to discern the activity resulting from each of the medications.

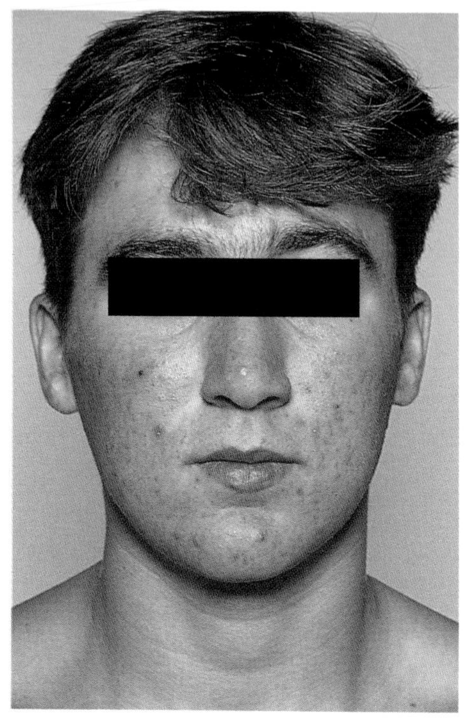

Figure 7.1

Superficial but inflamed acne.

For the reasons given above, the use of topical tretinoin together with other topical medication is to be discouraged, unless they are pharmaceutically prepared as a single topical application. A case can be made for concurrent use of an antibacterial application such as topical benzoyl peroxide or one of the topical antibiotics, but these should be used at a different time of the day. The dangers of inactivation of the tretinoin are minimized if the tretinoin is given at night and the other agent is used in the morning. Another approach is to use each of the topical agents on alternate days.

What concentration of tretinoin and which type of vehicle should be given initially? This is a matter of experience and judgement and will in part depend on the tolerance of the patient as well as the severity of the acne present. In general, the gel formulations tend to evoke a more vigorous response. Fair-complexioned individuals respond to lower concentrations and may not be able to tolerate the higher concentrations, and lower concentrations need to be used in the winter when the skin is more sensitive. Usually patients with mild to moderately severe superficial acne with a moderate number of comedones and a few inflamed papules and pustules respond best to topical tretinoin. These patients would be categorized as having grades 1–3 inclusive in Cunliffe's scheme.[1] Patients with deep papules, nodules and cysts should have other forms of treatment, although such patients may benefit from topical tretinoin if they have a superficial component in addition. Furthermore, use of topical tretinoin may prevent deep inflamed lesions.

Most patients respond within 3–4 weeks to once daily application of the topical tretinoin with a reduction in the numbers of comedones and papules.[2–4] There is perhaps a 60–70 per cent improvement in the acne in up to 70 per cent of patients with superficial and comedonal acne. There is also very considerable improvement in elderly patients with so-called senile comedones.[5]

Side-effects from the use of topical tretinoin

Virtually all patients who use topical tretinoin experience some dryness and scaling of the treated areas. In addition, the areas become pink. Very few patients find that they are unable to tolerate the minor discomfort and soreness that this causes. It has to be remembered that many of the other topical preparations used for acne also have a slight irritative effect. Sulfur and benzoyl peroxide are well known to produce dryness and scaliness. In addition, benzoyl peroxide can uncommonly cause allergic contact dermatitis[6] which is not a problem with tretinoin.

Many youngsters who use tretinoin preparations for their acne notice that they become more sensitive to the sun and may sunburn more easily than before starting treatment. This does not appear to be a true photochemical reaction in which the drug and UVR interact to cause a toxic dermatitis, or a true photoallergic sensitization. Rather it seems that although the epidermis thickens (see below) the stratum corneum of tretinoin-treated skin becomes somewhat thinner owing to enhanced desquamation. The thinner stratum corneum does not provide as much photoprotection as the normal stratum corneum and UVR damage readily occurs. For this reason, if for no other, it is advisable to prescribe a sunscreen for patients on topical tretinoin. Patients should, of course, be warned about both the slight soreness and scaling that they will develop as well as the increased sensitivity to the sun.

Because of this increased sensitivity to the sun there has been some concern over the possible photocarcinogenic potential of topical tretinoin. There has been some support for this concern in that UV-irradiated mice that were also being treated topically with tretinoin developed more skin cancers compared with controls.[7] This result, however, has to be considered in the context of the following: (a) numerous similar experiments have been reported that do not suggest a photocarcinogenic potential; (b) the anticancer effects of the retinoids (see chapter 8) are well known and topical tretinoin itself has been used to treat solar keratoses;[8] and (c) there have been no reports of an excess of skin cancers in groups of patients using tretinoin for acne compared with others not so treated.

Another worry over the use of topical tretinoin is that it may have a teratogenic effect. There is no doubt that the retinoic group of drugs (including vitamin A) are potent teratogens. Although this is the case too with tretinoin, it does not appear likely that sufficient will be absorbed after topical application to a limited area of skin to present an appreciable risk. Indeed, in experiments in which topical tretinoin was applied with occlusion to 30 per cent of the body surface of human volunteer subjects, the blood levels of tretinoin did not increase above the normal levels found (tretinoin is a normal metabolite of vitamin A). In addition, there is no clinical evidence of an increased number of fetal malformations associated with maternal use of the preparation during early pregnancy. For example, no excess abnormalities were found in fetuses of women who had used topical tretinoin within a few months of conception compared with those women who had not been exposed to tretinoin during pregnancy.[9] Even though there is no evidence of any hazard to the unborn child, it is probably prudent not to prescribe preparations containing tretinoin for pregnant women or women who are trying to become pregnant.

Other topical retinoids in the treatment of acne

Isotretinoin (13-*cis*-retinoic acid), the *cis*-isomer of tretinoin, is the orally administered drug that has proved so successful in the treatment of the more severe forms of acne (see below). Because of its success as an oral agent it was natural to question whether it would also be useful when applied topically. Isotretinoin, like tretinoin, is tricky to formulate for topical use because of its instability and tendency to photodegradation. However, stable gel preparations of isotretinoin have been produced and appear active when applied to the skin. A topical formulation of 0.1% isotretinoin is licensed for use in acne and is proving popular and effective. The available published studies confirm that the preparation does indeed have therapeutic activity. For example, the study by Chalker et al has shown a clear advantage of the isotretinoin gel over an unmedicated identical placebo gel at 5 weeks and a continuing improvement after that time.[10] It has also been claimed that, at least on an equivalent concentration basis, topical isotretinoin is less irritant than topical tretinoin.

Other studies have shown that isotretinoin 0.05% gel reduced both inflamed and non-inflamed lesions, and has approximately the same therapeutic activity as 5% benzoyl peroxide.[11]

Another topical retinoid that has been used in the treatment of acne is motretinide. This compound certainly has similar stimulatory activity to tretinoin on the epidermis, causing similar degrees of epidermal thickening, increases in epidermal proliferation as judged by tritiated thymidine autoradiographic labelling indices, and acceleration of desquamation.[12] However, anecdotal reports suggest that its therapeutic activity is somewhat limited and certainly less than that of topical tretinoin.

Two other topical retinoids will be mentioned here. The first of these is a novel naphthalenic retinoid known as Adapalene (CD 271). When a 0.1% gel of Adapalene was compared with tretinoin 0.025% gel in a randomized double-blind trial in 323 acne patients, the Adapalene was significantly more effective and better tolerated[13] than tretinoin 0.025%. This is now licensed for the treatment of acne in several countries. The other new retinoid agent is AGN190168 or tarzarotene. This is a novel acetylenic retinoid that is receptor selective and was developed primarily for use in psoriasis (see Chapter 6). It has also been submitted to clinical trials in acne and the gel preparations used found to be effective for this purpose.

Mode of action of topical retinoids

To have a therapeutic effect in acne, a drug should suppress the rate of sebum flow, reduce the bacterial flora in the follicular canal, promote drainage from the follicle by loosening comedones (comedolysis) or have an anti-inflammatory effect. Topical tretinoin does not seem to reduce sebum production; although it was previously claimed that topical isotretinoin did have such an action, it is now generally agreed that this is not the case.[14] The major action of topical tretinoin is in causing epidermal hyperproliferation and an increase in the rate of desquamation.[12,15] This appears to result in shedding of the comedones and presumably in enhanced drainage from the follicular mouths. Whether this is the entire story or not is impossible to say at the moment, but the enormous amount of research on the retinoids currently under way suggests that we may have a clearer view on this issue in the near future.

Treatment of acne with systemic retinoids

The use of orally administered isotretinoin has transformed the management of patients with severe acne. As with many real therapeutic advances, the beneficial effect of isotretinoin was noted serendipitously. Peck and co-workers[16] found, during the experimental treatment of young patients with lamellar ichthyosis who incidentally had cystic acne, that their acne also improved. This group subsequently showed that 13 of 14 patients with severe nodulocystic acne cleared within 4 months of starting treatment with 2 mg/kg per day and, even more remarkably, stayed clear for long periods. No other retinoid has been found to cause the same dramatic improvement, although it was noted that large doses of vitamin A by mouth did have some therapeutic effects.[17,18]

Kligman et al investigated the issue more recently.[19] In this study, in which 300 000 i.u. vitamin A was given daily, vitamin A did not appear to have the same effect quantitatively on sebum secretion rate as does oral isotretinoin, as reductions of only about 29 per cent were found. However, the regimen used proved quite successful, resulting in a greater than 50 per cent improvement in 70 of the 80 men and 55 of the 56 women treated. They found that, at the dose level they used for a period not exceeding 3 months, the mucosal side-effects were similar to those observed with other oral retinoids, but hyperlipidaemia and abnormal liver tests were more frequently observed. They noted that 'accommodation to the toxic side effects occurred', and suggested that 'retinol has a definite place for the treatment of inflammatory acne'. Interestingly, the authors noted that relapse occurred a few months after the course of treatment – rather than the much longer periods found with isotretinoin (see below). As noted above, vitamin A does produce some reduction in sebum secretion rate but it is not known whether this is its prime mode of action or not.

It is important to note that not all have found that vitamin A has any improving effect in acne.[20] Our view is that there can be few patients for whom the drug is really useful, as vitamin A in 'therapeutic doses' seems to have somewhat greater toxicity and markedly less efficacy than isotretinoin, and for all practical purposes it need not be considered further as a useful treatment for acne.

Etretinate has also been studied to determine whether it has any beneficial effect in acne. Interestingly, it seems to have very much less therapeutic effect than isotretinoin, but this assertion is based on the results of a study of only ten patients which lasted for 8 weeks only, during which time there was an average reduction in the number of lesions of 30 per cent.[21] The reason why isotretinoin is so dramatically successful compared to etretinate has not been discovered. The literature is remarkably silent on this issue, which is sad, as this difference between the two drugs may hold important messages both for the way isotretinoin works and for the pathogenesis of acne.

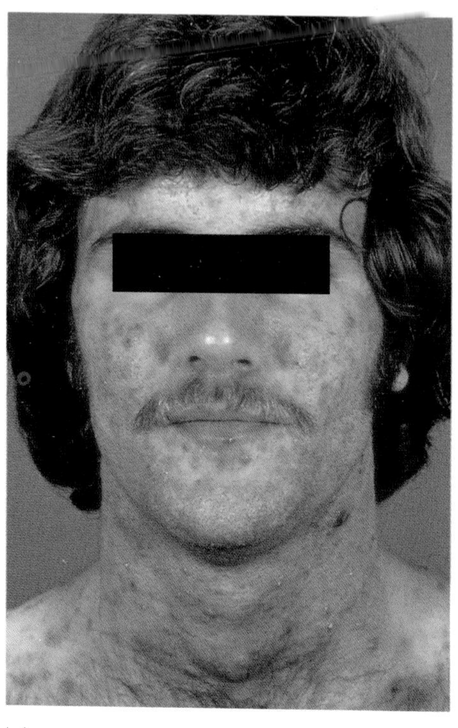

(a)

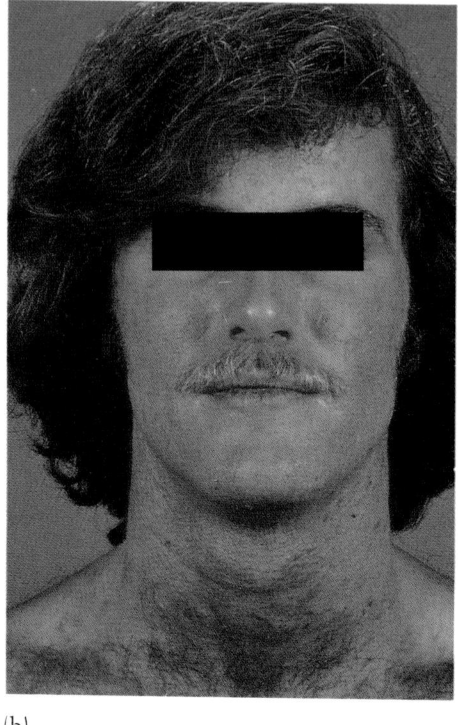

(b)

Figure 7.2

Severe nodulocystic acne: **(a)** before and **(b)** after treatment with oral isotretinoin 1 mg/kg per day for 5 months. (Courtesy of NJ Lowe, MD.)

The use of systemic isotretinoin for acne

Indications

Isotretinoin was originally prescribed only for patients with severe acne, with multiple cystic lesions and/or deep papules and papulonodules, and was restricted to this group because of the toxicity of the drug (see below). Those acne sufferers with numerous deep and inflamed lesions, who have proved resistant to all other forms of treatment affecting several sites, also qualify for this form of treatment. This should not mean that no other type of patient should ever be considered for isotretinoin. Indeed, in recent years views have changed, and some patients with only moderately severe but recalcitrant acne are now also treated with isotretinoin. As with most potent drugs, all factors have to be taken into consideration before a decision as to whether or not to treat is

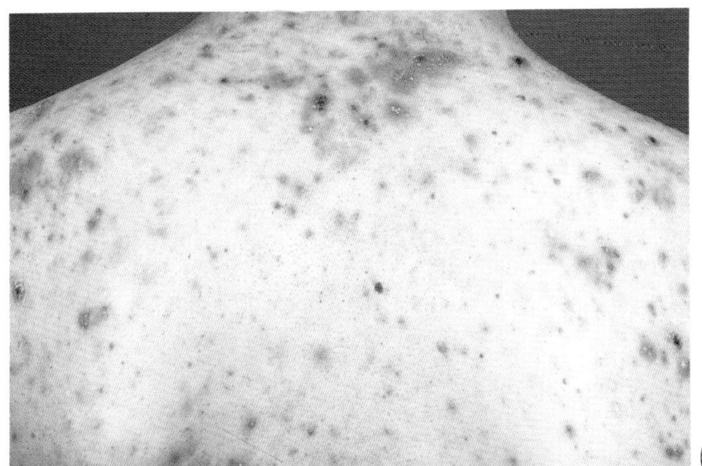

(a)

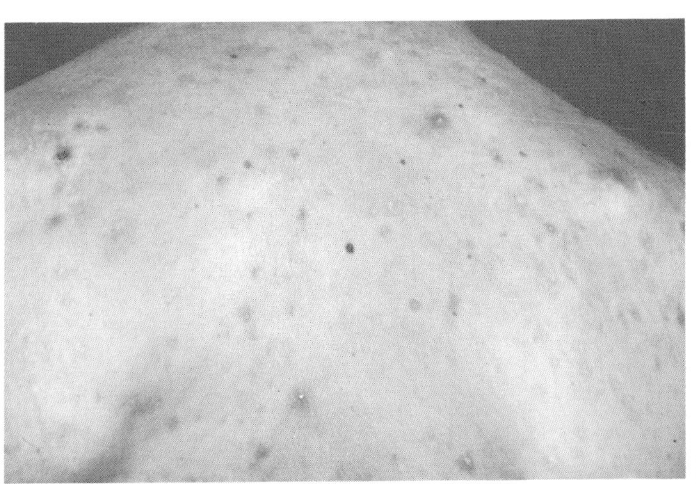

(b)

Figure 7.3

Severe acne: (**a**) before and (**b**) after treatment with oral isotretinoin 1 mg/kg per day for 5 months. (Courtesy of NJ Lowe, MD.)

taken. Certainly a major consideration is the profound improvement that patients experience (Figures 7.2–7.5).

Clearly, the degree of disability will influence the decision. A young man who is becoming severely depressed because of moderately severe acne over his face and shoulders may welll be a suitable recipient of the drug if all else has failed. On the other hand, a 'macho' type of youth who has proved to be unreliable with regard to clinic attendance and in taking previously prescribed medication as directed is probably a poor candidate, even though he has quite extensive and severe acne.

Young women in the reproductive age group pose a particular problem because of the teratogenicity of the drug (see below). If it is felt that, all other things being equal, the young woman would greatly benefit from having isotretinoin, then the first obligation of the physician is to ensure that the patient understands the side-effects, and the risks of

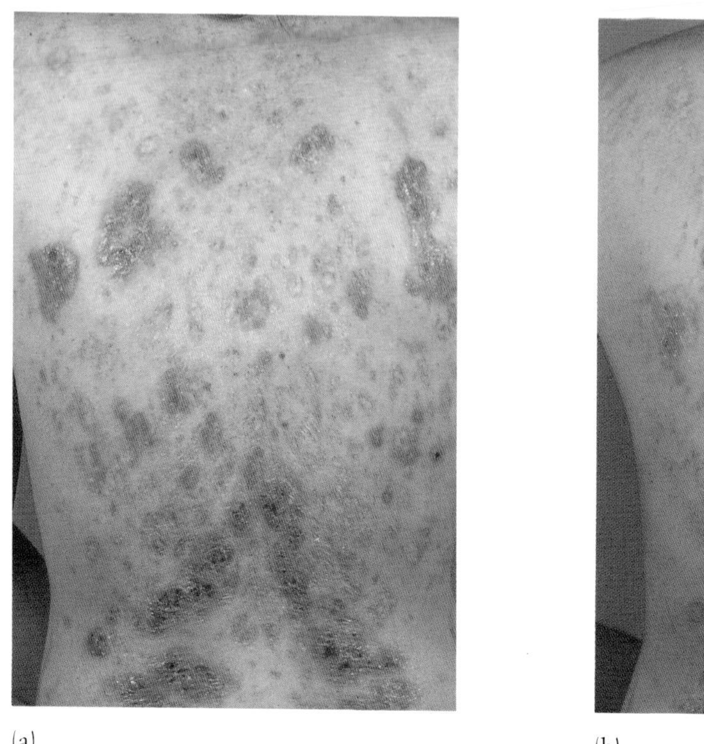

(a)

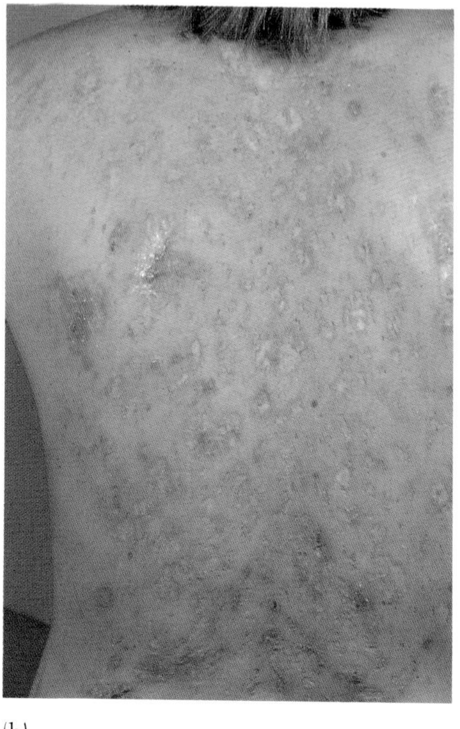

(b)

Figure 7.4

Severe acne of back: **(a)** before and **(b)** after treatment with oral isotretinoin 1 mg/kg per day for 5 months. (Courtesy of NJ Lowe, MD.)

serious toxicity, as well as the potential benefits. The next issue concerns contraception. It is the view of the author that the drug should not be prescribed for women in the reproductive age range who do not understand the issue involved and cannot or will not give a signed undertaking to the effect that they are using an efficient form of contraception. It is also required that the patient agrees that should she become pregnant while on the drug she will voluntarily seek a termination of pregnancy. Such 'heavy measures' have become necessary not only to protect the individual patient (and physician) but to ensure that regulatory bodies continue to allow the drug to be used at all.

The other factors that have to be considered when deciding whether or not to prescribe isotretinoin include the ability of the individual to return to the clinic at regular intervals for periods of 6 months or more. It is important to be able to check on the progress of the patient and on the development of side-effects and toxicities during the period of treatment.

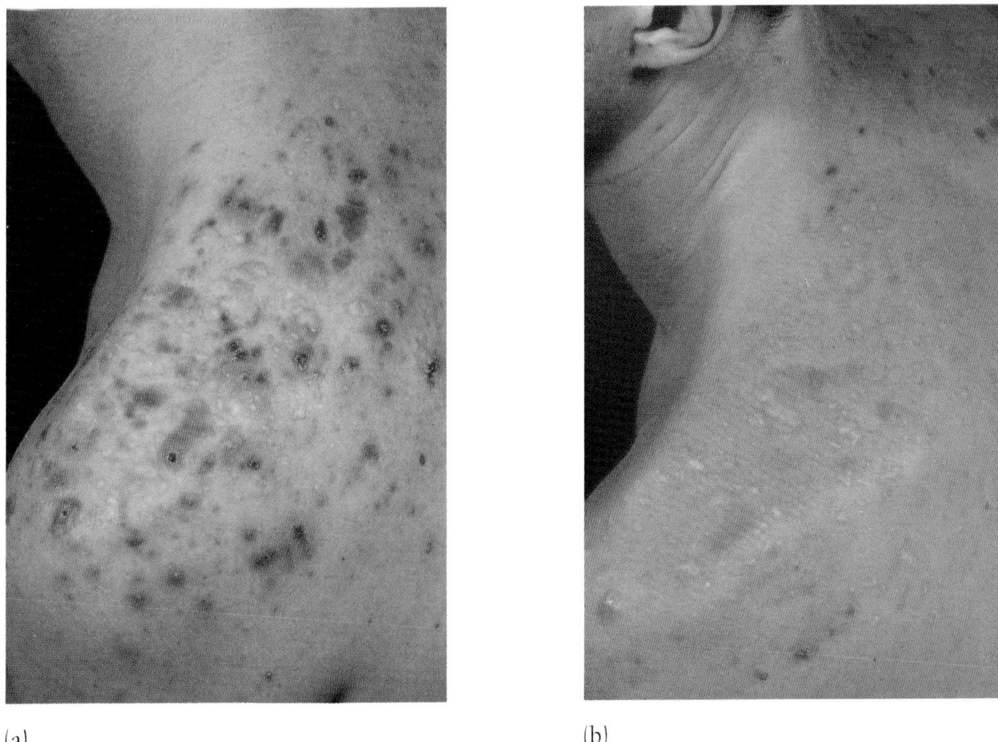

Figure 7.5

Improvement in acne: **(a)** before and **(b)** after treatment with oral isotretinoin 1 mg/kg per day for 5 months. (Courtesy of NJ Lowe, MD.)

Pre-existing hyperlipidaemia or hepatic or bone disease will also influence the decision as to whether or not to treat with isotretinoin. The influence that concomitant disease and its treatment has on the use of isotretinoin has been studied by the Leeds group,[22] and it is clear that intercurrent disease is not a proper reason for withholding treatment with isotretinoin.

Goulden et al[23] of the Leeds group state 'our study shows that the indications for isotretinoin have significantly altered over the past several years. They now include as indications partial response to conventional treatment and a predominant facial distribution'.

Last, and by no means least, is the financial implication of prescribing isotretinoin. The cost of providing isotretinoin in the United Kingdom at a dose of 1 mg/kg per day for a notional 70-kg man for a 16-week period may be of no consequence for the son or daughter of an affluent middle-class family, but it has come to be an issue in the impoverished UK National Health Service and in

Table 7.1 **Factors influencing prescription of isotretinoin for acne**

Factor	*Comment*
Severity of acne	Nodulocystic of one or more sites Severe extensive deep papular acne Other forms of disabling acne
Response to other treatments	Lack of or inadequate response to full doses of systemic antibiotics
Compliance and reliability	Patient can and will return to clinic
Comprehension	Patient understands toxicities and need for regular visits
Sex	Female patients *must not* be pregnant at start of treatment and *must* take reliable contraceptive measures before starting *and* must agree to termination if they become pregnant during treatment or within 1 month after stopping

countries where medical services are financed by a not-so-wealthy state. There is no perfect answer to this problem – but one can say that drugs have to be paid for and it is hoped that those who administer the medical budgets recognize that the drug is not prescribed without considerable thought, and that it certainly provides immense therapeutic benefit. There is strong economic argument for the use of isotretinoin: it has been computed that its use saves money in the long run as the patients improve relatively quickly and need much less in the way of other forms of treatment.[24]

The factors that influence whether or not isotretinoin is prescribed are set out in Table 7.1

Dosage and length of treatment

There have been several studies that have investigated the effects of different doses of isotretinoin.[25–30] The usual dose is between 0.5 and 1 mg/kg body weight per day. Certainly there does not seem to be additional benefit from the use of higher doses of 1.5 or 2.0 mg/kg per day, although the toxicities increase. Doses of 0.1 and 0.5 mg/kg per day have also been shown to be effective therapeutically, but doses below 0.5 mg/kg per day have also been shown to be associated with a higher relapse rate and a shorter time to relapse. The drug is quite water soluble and its absorption is not much influenced by food. None the less it is reasonable to ask that the drug is taken with food. It is customary to give the drug twice daily so as to maintain therapeutic concentrations in the blood. Isotretinoin is for the most part cleared from the body 1 month after ceasing treatment.

Treatment in an initial course is usually for a period of 16 weeks. It is worth noting that improvement often continues after the 16-week period for a further 4–8 weeks. If remission has not been obtained after this it seems agreed that it is best to give a 'treatment holiday' of 4–6 weeks before recommencing for a further 16-week treatment course. Some flare-up of the condition occurs in 20–30 per cent of patients treated with isotretinoin between 2 and 4 weeks after starting treatment. In this group of patients more lesions of all types appear, particularly pustules which may suddenly appear in large numbers. The existing lesions also become more inflamed. Improvement starts to take place at between 6 and 8 weeks and continues to about 12 weeks, after which further improvement is much slower.

Response to isotretinoin

Most studies show an improvement of approximately 80 per cent after a 16-week course of treatment. Layton and Cunliffe[31] report a 61 per cent 'cure rate', implying that these patients are not troubled again. Several studies have found that patients with severe truncal acne respond less well than patients with facial lesions only.[28,30] Overall, some 80 per cent of patients show something approaching an 80 per cent improvement in their condition. A substantial proportion of patients who do not show a good response to the first 16-week course of treatment show a gratifying response to the second course.[29] In one study[32] 94 per cent of patients treated with either 1.0 or 0.5 mg/kg per day showed a 'successful' response, 13 per cent had residual lesions and needed a second 16-week course to clear their acne, and some 8 per cent were resistant to treatment. Further courses may be given, but the risk of bone toxicity may start to become appreciable if treatment is continued for long periods, and anyway there may be other reasons (such as non-compliance) why these patients are not responding.

Unlike other forms of treatment for acne the remission that is induced by isotretinoin is long-lasting. As mentioned above, often no further treatment is required. For example, in the study of Jones and Cunliffe[30] 53 per cent maintained improvement for 28 weeks post-treatment, while 44 per cent remained in remission for up to 2 years after treatment. However, relapses become more frequent the longer the period that has elapsed from stopping treatment. Interestingly, although the rate of sebum secretion may stay suppressed (see below) for up to a year following cessation of treatment, it usually does return to the pre-treatment level (Figure 7.6). Although sebum secretion does eventually return to its previous level the acne does not necessarily accompany the resurgence of activity of the sebaceous glands. Relapse appears much more frequently in those patients who have been given less than 0.5 mg/kg per day for periods of less than 16 weeks. Thus, although 87 per cent of patients treated with 0.1 mg/kg per day showed a good response, only 23 per cent remained in remission for 28 weeks, and only 5 per cent remained free of acne for 2 years. There even appears to be a benefit from 1.0 mg compared with 0.5 mg/kg per day with regard to prolonged remission, as it has been found that there was a worse relapse rate in the 0.5 mg/kg per day group than in the 1.0 mg/kg per day group.[30–32]

Side-effects and toxicities

Isotretinoin is associated with a high incidence of a number of minor annoying side-effects and is almost exactly identical to etretinate in this respect. The most common of these, occurring in more than 90 per cent of patients, is a characteristic cheilitis. The lips become dry, scaly and cracked, and may be the cause of considerable discomfort. Other mucosal or 'transitional' areas may also become dry and uncomfortable. Facial dermatitis is mentioned by some authors as a troublesome side-effect in approximately 25–30 per cent but it is much less common in

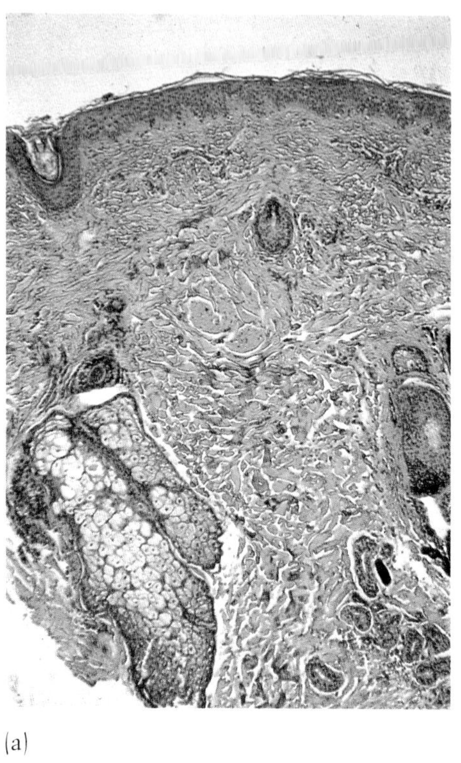

(a)

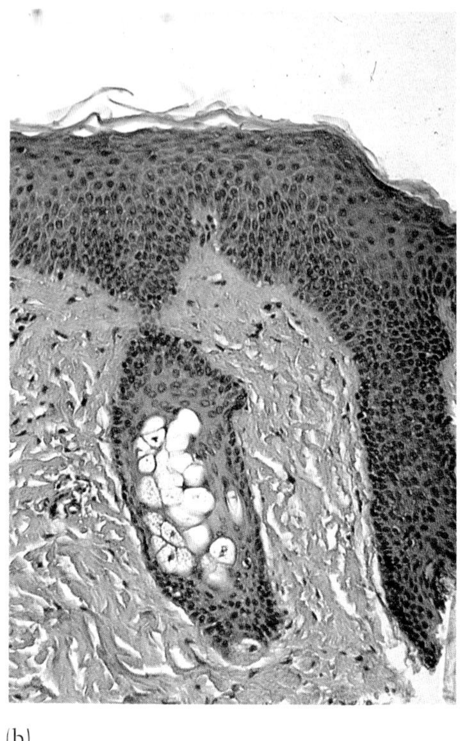

(b)

Figure 7.6

Skin biopsies taken **(a)** before and **(b)** after oral isotretinoin therapy 1 mg/kg per day for 5 months (upper back skin). (Courtesy of NJ Lowe, MD.)

this author's experience. A few patients complain of a 'dry mouth' but serious drying of the buccal mucosa does not seem to occur. The eyes occasionally feel dry and gritty and in one study,[33] conducted in Austria, some 69 per cent of 55 patients showed a pathological decrease of tear break-up time and 40 per cent had blepharitis. These authors also cultured *Staphylococcus aureus* from the conjunctival sacs of 61.8 per cent of patients on isotretinoin compared with 7.3 per cent before starting treatment. Drying of the nasal mucosa is sometimes quite troublesome. In approximately 15 per cent of patients it leads to bleeding from the nasal mucosa. The anogenital mucosa may also show some dryness but this is not usually troublesome. Slight soreness and peeling of the palms and soles are seen in approximately 10–15 per cent of patients using isotretinoin, but once again this is not usually the cause of serious complaint.

Of more significance, as far as the patient is concerned, is the increased hair fall. This rarely results in a significant cosmetic disability and is anyway transitory, lasting only while the patient is on the drug. It is none the less frequently a cause of considerable anxiety. The exact cause of this is uncertain but is not an anagen effluvium as it would be with a cytostatic agent.[34]

Musculoskeletal side-effects were recognized some years after the drug was first introduced. Strauss et al[28] found that limb and joint pain were dose related, being found in 18 per cent of patients on 0.5 mg/kg per day but in 30 per cent on 1.0 mg/kg per day. The relationship of these symptoms to the development of radiological changes in the bony skeleton is uncertain.

Apart from these relatively minor side-effects, isotretinoin is capable of causing serious and potentially irreversible toxic effects. These are teratogenicity,[35] bone toxicity (including ossification of tendons and ligaments),[36–40] liver toxicity,[41] pseudomotor cerebri[42] and hyperlipidaemia.[43–45] While these effects are seen mainly on patients on long-term retinoid treatment and are not often a problem in practice, every dermatologist who prescribes isotretinoin must know and understand them. The more severe toxicities are described fully in chapter 10.

Treatment of acne-related disorders

Treatment of rosacea with retinoids

Rosacea appears to be a fundamentally different disorder to acne and should not be regarded as a type of adult acne. For the majority of patients the established treatment of the condition with tetracycline or erythromycin is sufficient at least to suppress the disfiguring papules and pustules that patients find so distressing. Metronidazole given either systemically or topically is also effective. However, the erythema that affects all rosacea patients is not helped much by these treatments and neither is the rhinophyma.

Rhinophyma appears to respond well to oral isotretinoin given in the same dosage but for longer periods than for acne (Figure 7.7). In one study the 'volume' of the noses of affected patients was measured using image analysis and a technique employing plaster casts before and after treatment. The nasal volume was significantly reduced at the end of the treatment period.[46] Other studies also attest as to the efficacy of this form of treatment.[47] Unfortunately there are as yet insufficient data to give a firm opinion concerning relapse rate, although clinical experience suggests that relapse may be anticipated within a few months of stopping treatment in most patients.

Surgical management of rhinophyma is so good these days that oral retinoids are not often called for in its treatment. None the less some patients may prefer this non-invasive approach.

Recently some thought has been given to the possibility of using topical retinoids for chronic erythema and telangiectasia. If, as the author believes, dermal disorganization from photodamage is the basis of the disorder and is responsible for the persistent erythema and telangiectasia, it is logical to believe that topical retinoids may ultimately help. Indeed, Kligman has documented such an improvement in a group of patients,[48] and this is the author's experience as well.

Hidradenitis suppurativa

This condition can be disabling, and the current best form of treatment is the surgical removal of all the affected apocrine-bearing skin, a technique pioneered by Hughes of Cardiff. However, some have claimed that oral isotretinoin improves the condition.[49]

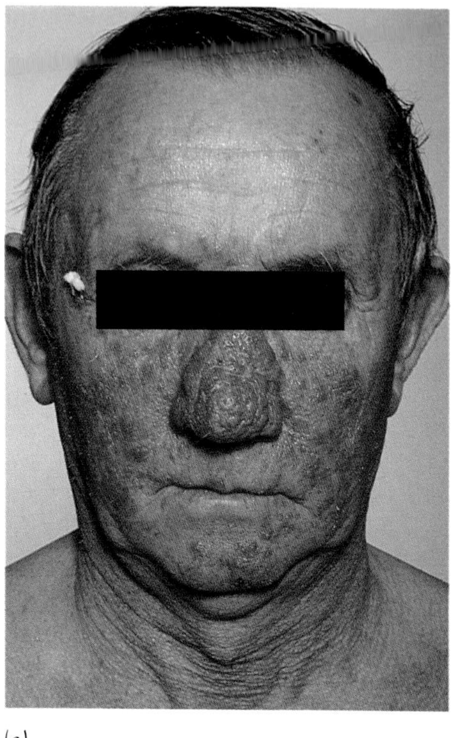

(a)

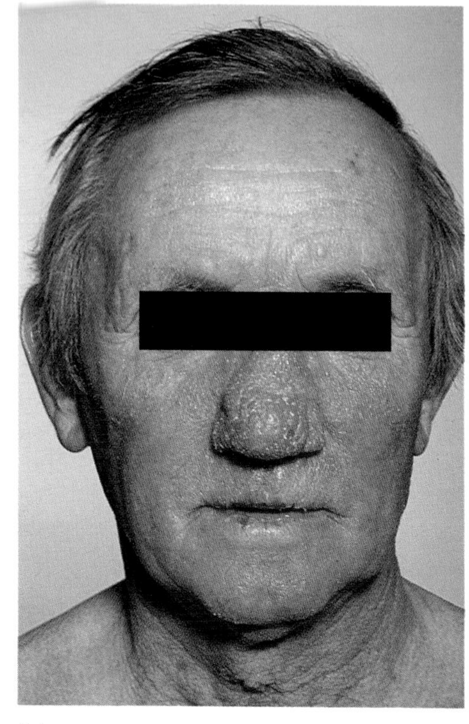

(b)

Figure 7.7

Rhinophyma **(a)** before and **(b)** after treatment with isotretinoin 1 mg/kg per day.

Our own experience with oral retinoids in hidradenitis has not been encouraging and in our view they should only be regarded as a 'last resort'.

References

1. Cunliffe WJ, Clinical assessment of acne vulgaris. In: Cunliffe WJ, (ed.). *Acne*. Martin Dunitz: London, 1989, pp 115–22.
2. Cunliffe WJ, Retinoic acid. In: Cunliffe WJ (ed.). *Acne*. Martin Dunitz: London, 1989, p 256.
3. Leyden JJ, Shalita AR, Rational therapy for acne vulgaris: an update on topical treatment. *J Am Acad Dermatol* (1986) **15**: 907–14.
4. Kligman AM, Fulton JE, Plewig G, Topical vitamin A acid in acne vulgaris. *Arch Dermatol* (1969) **99**: 469–72.
5. Cunliffe WJ, Senile (solar) comedones. In: Cunliffe WJ (ed.). *Acne*, Martin Dunitz: London, 1989, p 60.
6. Cronin E, *Contact dermatitis*. Churchill Livingstone: London & Edinburgh, 1980, p 181.
7. Epstein JH, Photocarcinogenesis and topical retinoids. In: Marks R (ed.). *Retinoids in cutaneous malignancy*. Blackwell Scientific Publications: Oxford, 1991, ch 12.

8. Kligman AM, Thorne EG, Topical therapy of actinic keratoses with tretinoin. In: Marks R (ed.). *Retinoids in cutaneous malignancy*. Blackwell Scientific Publications: Oxford, 1991, ch 4.
9. Jick SS, Teris BZ, Jick H, First trimester topical tretinoin and congenital disorders. *Lancet* (1993) **341**: 1181–2.
10. Chalker DK, Lesher JL, Graham Smith J et al, Efficacy of topical isotretinoin 0.05% gel in acne vulgaris: results of a multicenter double blind investigation. *J Am Acad Dermatol* (1987) **2**(1): 251–4.
11. Hughes BR, Norris JFB, Cunliffe WJ, A double-blind evaluation of topical isotretinoin 0.05%, benzoyl peroxide gel 5% and placebo in patients with acne. *Clin Exp Dermatol* (1992) **17**: 165–8.
12. Marks R, Pearse AD, Black D et al, Techniques for assessing the activity of topically applied retinoids. *J Am Acad Dermatol* (1986) **15**(4/2): 810–16.
13. Shalita A, Weiss JS, Chalker DK et al, A comparison of the efficacy and safety of adapalene gel 0.1% and tretinoin gel 0.025% in the treatment of acne vulgaris: A multicenter trial. *J Am Acad Dermatol* (1996) **34**: 482–5.
14. Plewig G, Ruhfus A, Kovexorn W, Sebum suppression after topical application of retinoid (Arotinoid and isotretinoin). *J Invest Dermatol* (1993) **80**: 357(abstr).
15. Cunliffe WJ, Retinoic acid. In: Cunliffe WJ (ed.). *Acne*. Martin Dunitz: London, 1989, p 256.
16. Peck GL, Olsen TG, Yoder FW et al, Prolonged remissions of cystic and conglobate acne with 13-cis retinoic acid. *N Eng J Med* (1979) **300**: 329–33.
17. Straumfjord JV, Vitamin A: its effects on acne. *Northwest Med* (1949) **42**: 219–25.
18. Davidson DM, Sobel AE, Aqueous vitamin A in acne vulgaris. *J Invest Dermatol* (1949) **12**: 221–8.
19. Kligman AM, Leyden JJ, Mills O, Oral vitamin A (Retinol) in acne vulgaris. In: Orfanos CE, Braun-Falco O, Farber EM et al (eds), *Retinoids. Advances in basic research and therapy*, Springer-Verlag: Berlin, 1981, pp 245–53.
20. Anderson JAD, Stokoe, IH, Vitamin A in acne vulgaris. *Br Med J* (1963) **2**: 294–6.
21. MacKie RM, Dick DC, A clinical trial of the use of Tigason (Ro10-9359) in male patients with severe acne vulgaris. In: Orfanos CE, Braun-Falco O, Farber EM et al (eds). *Retinoids: Advances in basic research and therapy*, Springer-Verlag: Berlin, 1981, pp 267–9.
22. Macdonald Hull S, Cunliffe WJ, The safety of isotretinoin in patients with acne and systemic diseases. *J Dermatol Treat* (1989) **1**: 35–7.
23. Goulden V, Layton AM, Cunliffe WJ, Current indications for isotretinoin as a treatment for acne vulgaris. *Dermatology* (1995) **190**: 284–27.
24. Cunliffe WJ, Gray JA, Macdonald-Hull S et al, Cost effectiveness of isotretinoin. *J Dermatol Treat* (1991) **1**: 285–7.
25. Jones DH, King K, Miller AJ et al, The dose-response relationship of sebum suppression to 13-cis-retinoic acid therapy in severe acne. *Br J Dermatol* (1983) **109**: 366–7.
26. Farrel LN, Strauss JS, Stranieri AM, The treatment of severe cystic acne with 13-*cis* retinoic acid. *J Am Acad Dermatol* (1980) **3**: 602–11.
27. Plewig G, Wagner A, Braun-Falco O, Oral treatment of severe forms of acne with 13-*cis* retinoic acid. *Münch Med Wschr* (1980) **122**(38): 1287–92.
28. Strauss JS, Rapini RP, Shalita AR et al, Isotretinoin therapy for acne: Results of a multicenter dose-response study. *J Am Acad Dermatol* (1984) **10**: 490–6.
29. Rapini RR, Konecky EA, Schillinger B et al, Effect of varying dosages of isotretinoin in nodulocystic acne. *J Invest Dermatol* (1983) **80**: 358.
30. Jones DH, Cunliffe WJ, Remission rates in acne patients treated with various doses of 13-*cis*-retinoic acid. *Br J Dermatol* (1984) **111**: 123–5.
31. Layton AM, Cunliffe WJ, Guidelines for optimal use of isotretinoin in acne. *J Am Acad Dermatol* (1992) **27**(2/2): S2–7.
32. Cunliffe WJ, Jones DH, Pritlove J et al, Long term benefit of isotretinoin in acne – clinical and laboratory studies. In: Saurat J (ed.). *Retinoids: New trends in research and therapy*. Karger: Basel, 1985, pp 242–51.
33. Egger SF, Huber-Spitzy V, Böhler K et al, Ocular side-effects associated with 13-*cis*-retinoic acid therapy for acne vulgaris: clinical features, alterations of tearfilm and conjunctival flora. *Acta Ophthalmol Scand* (1995) **73**: 355–7.

34. Berth-Jones J, Shuttleworth D, Hutchinson PE, A study of etretinate alopecia. *Br J Dermatol* (1990) **122**: 751–6.
35. Sulik KK, Alles AJ, Teratogenicity of the retinoids. In: Saurat J-H (ed.). *Retinoids: 10 years on*, Karger: Basel, 1991, pp 282–95.
36. Pittsley RA, Yoder FW, Skeletal toxicity associated with long term administration of 13-*cis*-retinoic acid for refractory ichthyosis. *N Engl J Med* (1983) **308**: 1012–14.
37. Resnick D, Nuvayama G, Radiographic and pathological features of spinal involvement in diffuse iodiopathic skeletal hyperstosis (DISH). *Diagnostic Radiol* (1976) **119**: 559–68.
38. Lawson JK, McGuire J, The spectrum of skeletal changes associated with long term administration of 13-*cis*-retinoic acid. *Skeletal Radiol* (1987) **16**: 91–7.
39. Milstone LM, McGuire J, Ablow RC, Premature epiphyseal closure in a child receiving oral 13-*cis*-retinoic acid. *J Am Acad Dermatol* (1982) **7**: 663–6.
40. Kilcoyne RF, Cope R, Cunningham W et al, Minimal spinal hyperostosis with low dose isotretinoin therapy. *Invest Radiol* (1986) **21**: 41–4.
41. Mills CM, Marks R, Adverse reactions to oral retinoids – an update. *Drug Safety* (1993) **9**: 280–90.
42. Griffin JP, A review of the literature on benign intracranial hypertension associated with medication. *Adverse Drug Reaction Toxicol Rev* (1992) **11**: 41–58.
43. Melnik B, Bros U, Plewig G, Atherogenic risk of isotretinoin and etretinate compared. In: Marks R, Plewig G (eds). *Acne and related disorders*. Martin Dunitz: London, 1989, pp 227–30.
44. Marsden JR, Lipid metabolism and retinoid therapy. *Pharmacol Ther* (1989) **40**(1): 55–65.
45. Gollnick H, Schwartzkopf W, Proschle W et al, Retinoids and blood lipids: an update and review. In: Saurat J (ed.). *Retinoids: New trends in research and therapy*. Karger: Basel, 1985, pp 445–60.
46. Irvine C, Kumar P, Marks P, Isotretinoin in the treatment of rosacea and rhinophyma. In: Marks R, Plewig G (eds). *Acne and related disorders*. Martin Dunitz: London, 1989, pp 301–6.
47. Rödder O, Plewig G, Rhinophyma and rosacea: combined treatment with isotretinoin and dermabrasion. In: Marks R, Plewig G (eds). *Acne and related disorders*. Martin Dunitz: London, 1989, pp 335–8.
48. Kligman AM, Topical tretinoin for rosacea: a preliminary report. *J Dermatol Treat* (1983) **4**: 71–3.
49. Plewig G, Steger M, Acne inversa (alias acne triad, acne tetrad or hidradenitis suppurativa). In: Marks R, Plewig G (eds). *Acne and related disorders*. Martin Dunitz: London, 1989, pp 345–58.

8 Skin cancer

Ronald Marks

Introduction

The prophylactic effect of dietary vitamin A (retinol) against the development of epithelial cancers of many different types has long been known and quite intensively investigated. Work in the 1920s established that dietary retinol deficiency caused squamous metaplasia of the salivary glands, trachea, and genitourinary and gastrointestinal tracts in small mammals.[1,2] Even at that time it was noted that these metaplastic changes resembled those seen in premalignant disease. Subsequently, it has been demonstrated in several experiments that retinol-deficient animals are more likely to develop cancers after exposure to chemical carcinogens.[3,4] Other studies have shown that retinol is also capable of inducing reversal of premalignant conditions both in mice[5] and in cell and organ culture.[6,7]

These effects of retinol seem to be dose related and neither species nor carcinogen specific. This being so, there has been considerable interest in the use of retinol for cancer prophylaxis in humans. Certainly the available data suggest that there is an association between serum levels of vitamin A and the incidence of gastrointestinal and bronchial malignant disease.[8,9] There has also been a study of the complex relationship between dietary intake and serum levels of vitamin A and the development of skin cancer, but the results of this study are not conclusive.[10]

When it was decided to develop the group of retinol analogues we now know as retinoids, the prime aim was to employ them as anticancer drugs. Indeed the model originally developed for screening retinoids was the mouse papilloma model. In this, the ability of the retinoid in question, delivered weekly intraperitoneally over 2 weeks, to decrease greatly (by 50 per cent) the papillomatous and carcinomatous lesions induced by twice weekly painting of the skin with dimethyl benzanthracene for some months, is contrasted with the toxicity.[11] Happily the therapeutic ratios derived from this animal model are predictive of their therapeutic activity in a variety of other disorders affecting the epidermis such as psoriasis and the ichthyotic diseases, as well as in neoplastic diseases of skin. As has already been pointed out, retinol has preventative properties for many epithelial malignancies. Retinol analogues have also proved therapeutically useful for non-epithelial malignant diseases. Melanoma and lymphoma will be mentioned later, but here it is worthwhile mentioning the effects of some retinoids in treating acute promyelocytic leukaemia.[12] Curiously, etretinate does not seem effective for this purpose – exemplifying the point that in this group of diseases there is some retinoid molecule specificity. To support this concept of specificity, the retinoid 4-hydroxyphenyl retinamide (fenretinide) which is concentrated in breast tissue, has been, and is being, used in studies of breast cancer prevention in women who have already had one carcinoma of the breast.[13]

It is not clear whether this specificity of action in neoplastic disease is the result of different distributions of the different nuclear retinoic acid receptors and selective affinity for one or another of these receptors.

The oral retinoid drugs have a significant therapeutic effect in the various forms of non-melanoma skin cancer and precancer, whether caused by persistent exposure to solar UVR, by human papilloma viruses, by genetic faults in DNA repair or by other metabolic abnormalities. Topical retinoids also have a useful suppressive effect on solar keratoses. Retinoid compounds have also been employed as sole treatment or as part of treatment regimens in the management of mycosis fungoides and malignant melanoma. Indeed in recent years it has been recognized that retinoid drugs in combination with cytokines may have dramatically enhanced efficacy in malignant disease compared with the individual compounds alone. These issues will be covered later in this chapter.

Solar keratoses and squamous cell skin cancer

Solar keratoses (SKs) are common lesions which are supposedly premalignant, but longitudinal studies suggest that there is a very low risk (perhaps <0.1 per cent) of any one particular lesion progressing to a frank squamous cell carcinoma.[14] None the less SKs are indications that a significant degree of solar damage has been sustained and that the epidermis has been 'initiated' and consequently may develop a frank carcinoma at any time. SKs were found in 54 per cent of the population over 40 years of age in Queensland, Australia,[15] and even in comparatively damp and sunless Wales approximately 20 per cent of the population of South Glamorgan over the age of 60 were found to have SKs.[16]

Apart from their significance with regard to solar damage, SKs are also cosmetically upsetting, 'get in the way', and are sometimes itchy and sore. Patients who have been exposed to the sun over long periods and/or are especially susceptible develop large numbers of these annoying excrescences and need treatment for them. Both systemic and topical retinoids have been used.

Topical tretinoin was first used for SKs in 1962 by Stuttgen[17] and subsequently Bollag and Ott reported a highly satisfactory response to preparations containing 0.05% of this drug.[18] A recent large multicentre study of topical tretinoin has confirmed that it does keep SKs at bay although at least 6 months is required before any effects are obvious (Table 8.1).[19] Solar keratoses have also been treated by oral retinoid drugs including isotretinoin, etretinate, acitretin and an arotinoid (Ro 13-6298). Moriarty et al[20] reported the first double-blind controlled study of an oral retinoid in patients with multiple SKs. The study was carried out in Ireland where, because of the light-complexioned population of predominantly Celtic ancestry, non-melanoma skin cancer and SKs are extremely common. They treated 50 patients with histologically proven SKs, more than half of whom had had a form of non-melanoma skin cancer previously. These patients received 25 mg etretinate or placebo three times daily for a 2-month period and at the end of the 2 months the patients were 'switched over'. According to the authors, some 84 per cent of the 44 patients who completed the study showed a very good response to the etretinate.

Table 8.1 **Results of an open study of 0.05% tretinoin cream in patients with multiple solar keratoses[20]**

	Duration of treatment (months)							
	6 (n = 93)		*9 (n = 88)*		*12 (n = 25)*		*15 (n = 24)*	
	Before	*After*	*Before*	*After*	*Before*	*After*	*Before*	*After*
Mean lesion count	11.2	8.9	11.2	7.9	14.4	8.84	14.0	7.4
Difference	2.22		3.35		5.52		6.6	
P value	0.001		≤0.001		0.003		0.001	
Mean lesion size (mm)	84.1	62.6	84.7	55.4	131.7	72.8	124.1	61.4
Difference	21.9		29.3		58.9		62.7	
P value	0.00		≤0.001		0.014		0.009	

Oral isotretinoin has also been employed to treat SKs. For example, Beretti and Grupper[21] treated five patients with multiple keratoses, three of whom had arsenical keratoses. They used a dose of 1 mg/kg per day for a 4- or 5-month period and claimed that '75 per cent' of the patients cleared. Unfortunately, there is no more precise evaluation of the patient responses in this report, as well as no follow-up data. This report is typical of many published at that time in omitting any form of quantitative, objective measurement of the effects of the retinoids or any observations on relapse rate after treatment had stopped. It is not easy to produce quantitative estimates of the degree of improvement, but a simple measurement of the number of lesions present or a measurement of the combined area of the solar keratoses at least provides an approach to the problem.

Part of the problem stems from the fact that all of an area of skin that bears solar keratoses is probably affected by solar injury and the epidermis shows both structural and functional characteristics of dysplasia (photodysplasia). When treated with effective chemotherapeutic remedies it is not uncommon for previously apparently normal areas of skin to develop new inflamed SK-like lesions suddenly because of the widespread abnormality of epidermis that exists. Clearly counts of lesions at this point in treatment will give quite a false and depressing idea of the clinical response of the patient. Luckily, this stage in the treatment is usually comparatively short-lived, but it does emphasize the need for serial observations during any trial treatment with any chemotherapeutic agent.

Similarly, it is easy to obtain an over-optimistic view of the efficacy of treatment if

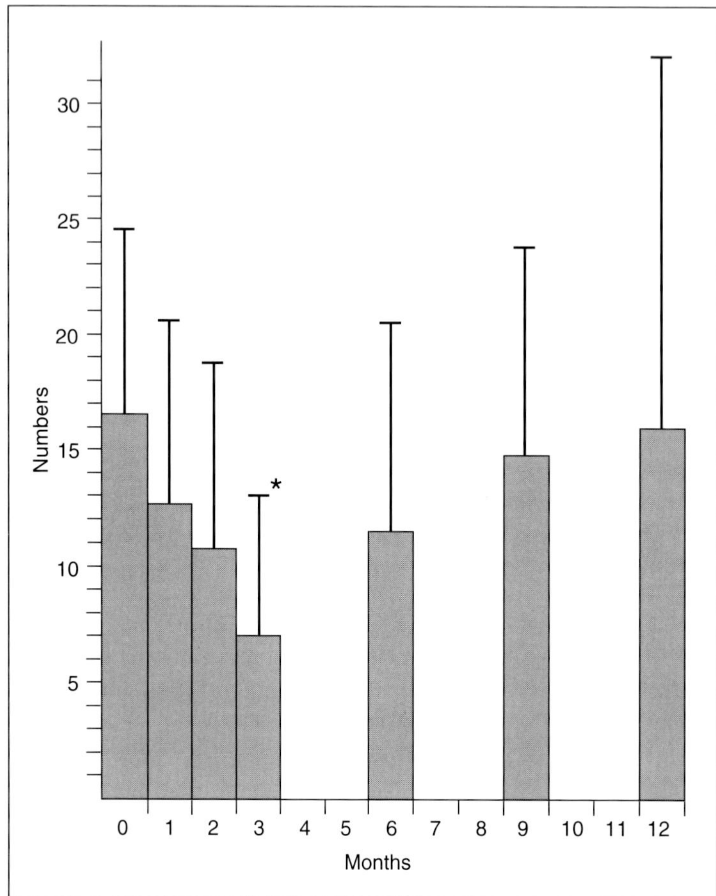

Figure 8.1

Therapeutic effect of acitretin 1 mg/kg per day on the mean number of solar keratoses in 12 patients as a function of time. *P = 0.002 (paired t-test).

patients are not followed up for sufficiently long periods. In one study performed in Cardiff in which acitretin was being evaluated,[22] although there was a striking reduction in the number of lesions in response to the drug in the first 3 months, during the 9 months that followed cessation of treatment the number of lesions increased to the pre-treatment levels (Figure 8.1).

A study by Hughes et al[23] demonstrated that both solar keratoses and basal cell carcinoma (BCC) respond to treatment with etretinate. A group of 15 patients was entered into this open-label study which lasted for 3 months with a follow-up period of 6–18 months. They were treated with etretinate 1.75 mg/kg per day for the first month but this was reduced to 0.75 mg/kg per day for the subsequent 2 months. Both types of lesion were significantly reduced at the end of the initial 3 months' treatment, but the solar keratoses were reduced more dramatically than the BCC (Table 8.2). Three patients with solar keratoses had no lesions at the 12-week assessment. Interestingly, five further patients became clear during the

Table 8.2 Mean number and area of solar keratoses and basal cell carcinoma in a study of effects of etretinate in non-melanoma skin cancer[23]

	Solar keratoses (12)		*Basal cell carcinoma (3)*	
	Mean no.	*Mean area (mm²)*	*Mean no.*	*Mean area (mm²)*
Pre-treatment	12.7	9.6	5.2	14.8
Post-treatment	5.8	3.2	3.8	12.9
Significance (*t*-test)	$P>0.005$	$P<0.005$	$P<0.05$	$P<0.01$

12 weeks after treatment stopped. Of the eight who cleared completely, only two developed recurrences (at 6 and 9 months) during the year in which they were observed.

This study by Hughes et al also revealed an important feature of the tissue response to the retinoid drug. Instead of there being a reduction in the epidermal proliferative activity, as one would expect from a cytostatic drug, there was a marked and significant increase in the tritiated thymidine autoradiographic labelling index in the post-treatment biopsies at all time points examined compared with the pre-treatment values. This increase in the labelling index signifies an increase in the rate of epidermal cell production. Not unnaturally, the increase was paralled by an increase in epidermal thickness (Tables 8.3a and 8.3b).

These results are quite similar to those found in an early study by Kingston et al,[24] in which the arotinoid Ro-13-6298 was used to treat patients with SKs and squamous cell carcinoma. Further confirmation of this effect was found in renal transplant recipients with SKs treated with etretinate.[25] Once again increased rather than decreased tritiated thymidine autoradiographic labelling indices were found in the skin of patients treated with etretinate. The same result was obtained when etretinate was administered to normal healthy volunteers.[26]

If, as seems to be the case, the systemically administered retinoids have a stimulatory effect on mitotic activity, how do they exert their antineoplastic effects? The answer to this important question is not available but it should not be thought that a cytostatic effect is a necessary property of an anti-cancer agent. Retinoids exert powerful actions on the way cells differentiate and it is possible that they direct dysplastic cells into more normal differentiating pathways and inhibit the neoplastic process in this way.

Some benefit for oral retinoids has been claimed in patients with advanced squamous cell carcinoma of the skin and it has also been claimed that isotretinoin inhibits the development of a second primary lesion.[27]

It is worth noting that a useful in vivo model has been developed in nude mice. Xenografts of human head and neck squamous carcinoma cells were implanted in the mice which were then treated with high doses of various retinoids. The xenografted tumour showed suppression of squamous differentiation but not always.[28]

Table 8.3a Effects of etretinate on tritiated thymidine autoradiographic labelling indices and mean epidermal thickness (MET) in lesional skin in patients with solar keratoses[23]

Time of second biopsy (week)	*MET (µm)*			*Labelling indices (%)*		
	No. patients	*Pre*	*Post*	*No. patients*	*Pre*	*Post*
2	2	107.7 (54.2–161.2)	241.5 (179.6–303.3)	2	9.6 (6.3–12.9)	19.2 (16.6–21.8)
4	3	70.65 (61.9–79.4)	158.1 (116.6–199.6)	2	13.7 (8.6–18.8)	15.9 (18.2–13.6)
8	2	73.0 (73.0)	98.3 (98.3)	2	6.3 (4.1–8.4)	16.7 (12.5–20.9)
12	2	103.5 (63.4–143.6)	99.6 (97.5–121.6)	2	8.5 (5.5–11.4)	12.6 (7.0–18.1)
Mean pooled data ± SD		91.0±43.0	156.6±77.9*		9.5±4.8	16.1±4.9*

*Significantly different from pre-treatment value.

Basal cell carcinoma

There have been several studies of the efficacy of retinoids in patients with multiple basal cell carcinoma. An early report[29] described the treatment of three patients with multiple BCC – one had the basal cell naevus syndrome (BCNS), one severe solar damage and the other a history of arsenic ingestion. Isotretinoin was given at a mean dose of 1.5 mg/kg per day for 4–6 months, and this was repeated after gaps of 1–2 months. The existing lesions showed a variable response in that only some regressed, but there was a dramatic prophylactic effect: no new lesions appeared over the ensuing 4 years. Peck et al[30] treated 12 patients with multiple BCC with different aetiologies. The patients were treated with a high mean dose of 3.1 mg/kg per day, but even this dose resulted in complete remission of only 8 per cent of the lesions. Lower doses (0.25–1.5 mg/kg per day) were found to be therapeutically ineffective but were effective in three of the patients. A particularly important subgroup of patients with BCC are those with BCNS. The report of Peck and co-workers does not mention specifically the results of treating the five patients who had BCNS, although the implication may be drawn from the report that the prophylactic effect of oral retinoids was not particularly dramatic in these individuals.

Table 8.3b **Effects of etretinate on tritiated thymidine autoradiographic labelling indices and mean epidermal thickness (MET) in uninvolved skin in patients with solar keratoses[23]**

Time of second biopsy (week)	*MET (μm)*			*Labelling indices (%)*		
	No. patients	*Pre*	*Post*	*No. patients*	*Pre*	*Post*
2	2	45.1 (43.9–46.3)	80.7 (76.2–85.2)	2	6.7 (6.2–7.1)	9.2 (10.7–7.6)
4	3	41.7 (31.5–57.6)	61.4 (57.1–65.1)	2	4.4 (4.0–4.8)	6.5 (6.3–6.7)
8	2	49.5 (43.2–55.7)	73.9 (44.9–102.8)	2	5.0 (4.9–5.1)	5.6 (5.6)
12	2	46.2 (39.4–52.9)	75.0 (46.2–103.8)	2	6.9 (3.2–10.5)	8.0 (8.0)
Mean pooled data ± SD		45.2±8.9	71.5±22.1*		5.8±2.3	7.6±1.6

*Significantly different from pre-treatment value.

The prophylactic effect was more obvious in a study by Goldberg et al[31] who treated twins with BCNS. Apparently before treatment both twins had 'hundreds of lesions'. One twin had 54 lesions removed between 1981 and 1982. A dose of isotretinoin of 0.4 mg/kg per day caused many lesions to disappear and inhibited the appearance of fresh lesions. One twin's dose was then reduced to 0.2 mg/kg per day while the dose of the other was maintained at twice this level. The difference was dramatic: the twin on the lower dose developed four times more new lesions than the twin on 0.4 mg/kg per day.

The response of BCCs to etretinate seems similar. There was only a modest response to etretinate (1.5 mg/kg per day for 1 month, then 1.0 mg/kg per day) in a study in Cardiff[23] (Table 8.2). Unfortunately low-dose prophylactic treatment with isotretinoin has not proved effective in preventing the development of new lesions of BCC. In a multicentre, randomized, double-blind study of the efficacy of 10 mg isotretinoin or placebo daily in 981 patients who had had two previous BCC lesions, no decrease in the number of new lesions was noted in the retinoid group compared with the placebo group over a 3-year period.[32] Despite this study it would certainly seem reasonable to try to inhibit the development of new lesions with a 'tolerable dose' of oral retinoids in patients with BCNS or those who regularly develop new BCC lesions from another cause.

Xeroderma pigmentosum and renal transplant patients

As intimated above with BCNS, clearly one major use for the retinoid drugs in the area of skin cancer is in patients with a large number of lesions who are continually liable to develop new ones. Xeroderma pigmentosum (XP) is such a group of patients. The defects in DNA repair in these individuals leads to numerous and varied skin cancers from an early age. There are several anecdotal reports of improvement in these unfortunate patients after treatment with oral retinoids, but understandably, few large studies have been carried out. Kraemer et al[33] treated seven patients with this condition with isotretinoin 2 mg/kg per day and demonstrated a considerable reduction in the numbers of new lesions that developed over a 2-year treatment period. Schnitzler[34] claimed a reduction in the number of new lesions in five patients treated with etretinate.

Etretinate was also helpful in the treatment of the six patients with multiple SK and squamous cell carcinoma (SCC) mentioned previously who had had renal transplants and were immunosuppressed (Figure 8.2).[25]

Acitretin has also proved helpful to renal transplant patients with keratoses and non-melanoma skin cancers. Twenty-four patients were treated with either acitretin 30 mg per day or a placebo, for a 6-month period. There was a relative decrease in the acitretin group of 13.4 per cent in keratotic lesions compared with an increase of 28.2 per cent in the placebo group.[35]

In an effort to reduce side-effects from oral retinoids, topical tretinoin was combined with etretinate daily in renal transplant patients. By 3 months of treatment, 9 of 11 patients showed at least a 25 per cent decrease in the number of neoplastic lesions.[36]

In epidermodysplasia verruciformis, numerous flat warty lesions develop over the limb and trunk skin owing to infection with human papilloma viruses (HPV) of different antigenic type, notably types 3 and 5. There appears to be an underlying immune deficit predisposing these individuals to the infection and to transformation of these warty lesions to SCC but this has not as yet been adequately characterized. Several groups have reported that oral etretinate improves such patients even though the viral particles persist (e.g. Jablonska et al,[37] Kanerva et al[38]). Warty dysplastic lesions on the feet, knees and elbows also occur in the Rothman–Thomson syndrome, and one such patient was treated successfully with etretinate in Cardiff.[39]

Mucosal lesions

Laryngeal papillomatosis is an odd and luckily uncommon disorder in which particular antigenic types of HPV cause warty lesions on the laryngeal mucosa of infants and young adults. Treatment has always been difficult and it is encouraging that three out of five patients with the condition who were treated with isotretinoin 0.5–2.0 mg/kg per day considerably improved.[40]

Cervical dysplasia has been treated by applications of tretinoin[41] but, at the time of writing, the long-term results are uncertain.

Leukoplakic lesions of the buccal mucosa have been treated with retinoids in several published studies. The first report is that of Cordero et al[42] who treated three patients with leukoplakia of the buccal mucosa and reported 'good' or 'excellent' results. Another study evaluated β-carotene (180 mg/week) and β-carotene with vitamin A (100 i.u./week) or placebo in a double-blind trial involving tobacco chewers in India. The

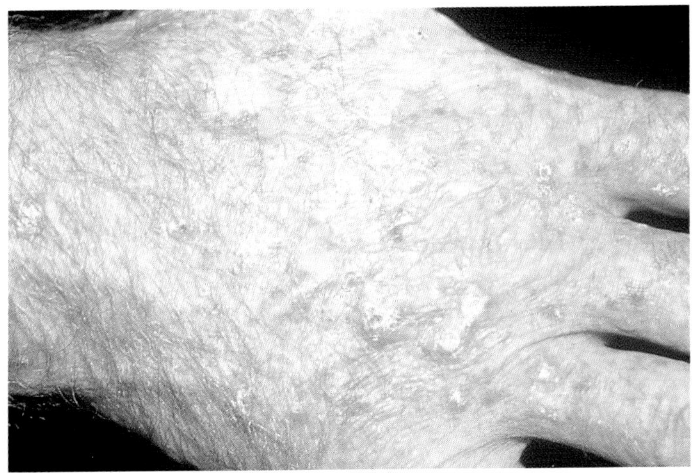

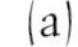

(a)

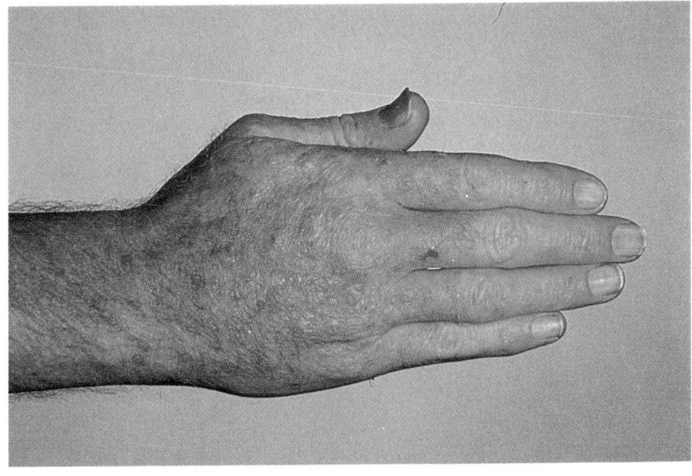

(b)

Figure 8.2

Solar keratoses on the back of the hand of a renal transplant patient treated with azathioprine and prednisone for 9 years: **(a)** before and **(b)** after treatment with etretinate. Most of the keratoses have disappeared or become smaller.

combined treatment group showed the greatest reduction in the appearance of new lesions (27.5 per cent) at 6 months compared with 14.8 per cent for the β-carotene group and 3.0 per cent for the placebo group.[43] A controlled study by Hong et al demonstrated that isotretinoin is quite successful in the treatment of oral leukoplakia.[44]

Although the bronchial mucosa is somewhat further than most dermatologists' reach, it is worth noting that retinoids have been used to try to improve the bronchial mucosal dysplasia of smokers. Two studies have been performed which regrettably have given contradictory results. The first claimed to demonstrate a reduction in the degree of bronchial metaplasia in patients treated with etretinate 25 mg/day over a 6-month period.[45] The more recent study performed in Canada was a complex placebo-controlled 6-month

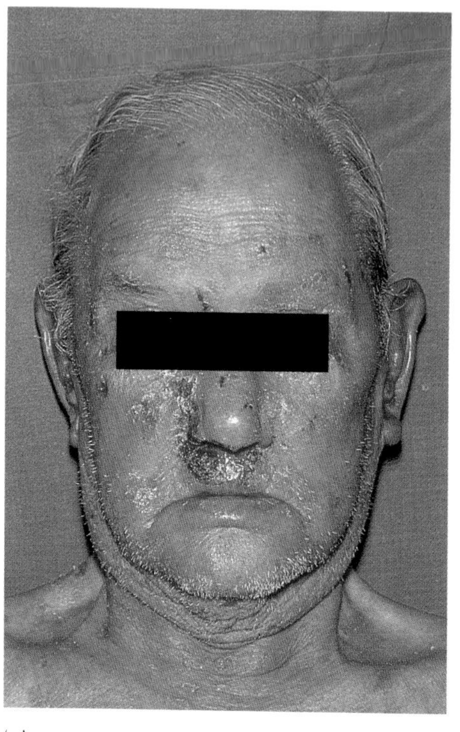

(a)

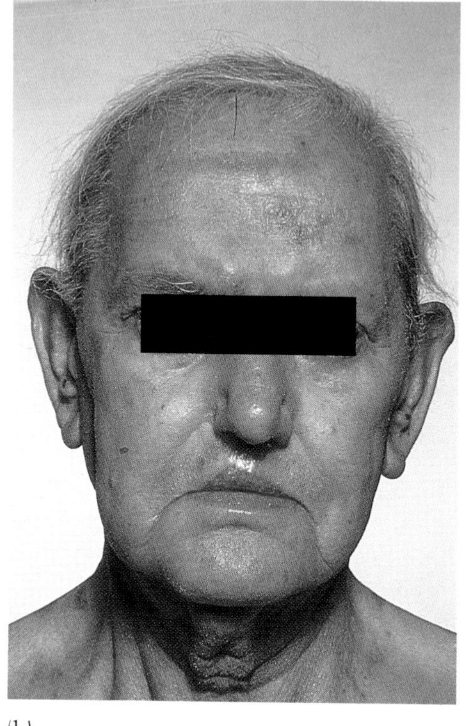

(b)

Figure 8.3

Patient with mycosis fungoides: **(a)** before and **(b)** after treatment with isotretinoin 1 mg/kg per day over a 6-week period. There was considerable improvement, but this patient died 3 months later.

study of 25 mg/day etretinate in which the sputum cytology was assessed blind.[46] No improvement in the degree of cellular atypia was detected in the etretinate treatment group.

Melanoma

Malignant melanoma is notoriously resistant to chemotherapy, but one patient with local metastases improved with topical tretinoin.[47] The combination of etretinate with interferon-alpha has also produced some limited benefit in patients with advanced malignant melanoma.[48] Although the retinoids do possess some therapeutic activity against melanoma, this form of treatment must be regarded as experimental and as a 'last ditch' effort to save a patient's life. Studies with melanoma cell lines show that some, but not all, are sensitive to retinoid drugs, and it is clear that this area of research is active and growing in importance. The subject is well reviewed by Lotan et al.[47] It should be noted that the use of topical tretinoin has resulted in a clinical and histological improvement in a significant number of dysplastic naevi treated with this agent.[52]

Lymphoma

The retinoids have been employed with or without comcomitant PUVA therapy in the treatment of mycosis fungoides (MF). Our own experience has been that isotretinoin (2 mg/kg per day) in particular can produce useful partial remissions (Figure 8.3). Claudy[49] reported that five of six patients with MF initially showed complete clinical clearing with etretinate 0.8–1.0 mg/kg per day for 2–24 months. A Scandinavian study reported that 19 of 28 patients showed good remissions with isotretinoin at initial doses of 2.0 mg/kg per day.[50] Another study on 25 patients[51] demonstrated a '44% objective clinical response rate' in a median time to response of 2 months and with a median response duration of 8 months (range 1–25 months). MF is always a difficult disease to treat, and sadly the ultimate result is always the same, but it does appear that clinically useful remissions can be induced with retinoid drugs.

Comment

The extensive literature leaves little doubt as to the antineoplastic actions of the retinoids. How they work is uncertain, but work they do. However, whether or not they are used for this purpose in a particular case will depend on the individual clinician and the particular clinical situation. Clearly there is no place for oral etretinate when there are two solar keratoses or a 'routine' BCC; their use here would be inappropriate. Similarly, when they cause serious toxic effects, as they do in high doses in some patients, they cannot be used. None the less, patients who have multiple SKs and/or many lesions of light-induced non-melanoma skin cancer, patients with XP or BCNS and those with MF are likely to benefit overall from this form of treatment.

References

1. Mori S, The changes in the paraocular glands which follow the administration of diets low in fat-soluble A with notes of the effects of the same diets on the salivary glands and the mucosa of the larynx and brachea. *Johns Hopkins Hosp Bull* (1922) **33**: 357–9.
2. Wolbach SD, Howe PR, Tissue changes following deprivation of fat-soluble A vitamin. *J Exp Med* (1925) **42**: 753–77.
3. Harris CC, Sporn MB, Kaufman DG et al, Histogenesis of squamous metaplasia in the hamster tracheal epithelium caused by vitamin A deficiency of benzo(a)pyrene ferric oxide. *J Natl Cancer Inst* (1972) **48**: 743–61.
4. Newberne PM, Rogers AE, Rat colon carcinomas associated with aflatoxin and marginal vitamin A. *J Natl Cancer Inst* (1973) **50**: 439–48.
5. Verma AK, Boutwell RK, Vitamin A acid (retinoic acid) a potent inhibitor of 12-O-tetradecanoyl-phorbol-13-acetate-induced ornithine decarboxylase activity in mouse epidermis. *Cancer Res* (1977) **37**: 2196–201.
6. Lasnitzki I, Goodman DS, Inhibition of the effects of methylcholanthrene on mouse prostate in organ culture by vitamin A and its analogs. *Cancer Res* (1974) **34**: 1564–71.
7. Harisiadis L, Miller RC, Hall EJ et al, A vitamin A analogue transformation. *Nature* (1978) **274**: 486–7.
8. Kark J, Smith A, Hames C, Serum retinol and inverse relationship between cholesterol and cancer. *Br Med J* (1982) **284**: 152–4.
9. Moon RC, Mehta RG, Vitamin A and the prevention of cancer. In: Marks R (ed.). *Retinoids in cutaneous malignancy*. Blackwell Scientific Publications: Oxford, 1991, pp 1–15.
10. Greenberg ER, Baron JA, Stukel TA et al, A clinical trial of beta carotene to prevent basal-cell and squamous-cell cancers of the skin. *N Engl J Med* (1990) **323**: 789–92.
11. Bollag W, Matter A, From vitamin A to retinoids in experimental and clinical oncology: achievements, failure and outlook. *Ann N Y Acad Sci* (1981) **359**: 9–23.
12. Jacobs A, Padua RA, Myelodysplasia and the retinoids. In: Marks R (ed.). *Retinoids in cutaneous malignancy*. Blackwell Scientific Publications: Oxford, 1991, pp 183–200.

13. Eliason JF, Teelmann K, Crettaz M, New retinoids and the future of the retinoids in the treatment of skin cancer. In: Marks R (ed.). *Retinoids in cutaneous malignancy*. Blackwell Scientific Publications: Oxford, 1991, pp 157–70.
14. Harvey I, Fraiker SJ, Shalom D et al, Non melanoma skin cancer: questions concerning its distribution and natural history. *Br Med J* (1989) **299**: 1118–20.
15. Green A, Beardmore G, Hart V et al, Skin cancer in a Queensland population. *J Am Acad Dermatol* (1988) **19**: 1045–52.
16. Shalom SD, Marks R, Harvey I, Sun exposure and solar damage in a Welsh population. In: Marks R, Plewig G (eds). *The environmental threat to the skin*. Martin Dunitz: London, 1992, pp 23–6.
17. Stüttgen G, Zur Lokalbehandlung der Keratosen mit Vitamin-A-Sure. *Dermatologica* (1962) **124**: 65–80.
18. Bollag W, Ott F, Retinoic acid: topical treatment of senile or actinic keratoses and basal cell cartinoma. *Agents Actions* (1970) **1**: 172–5.
19. Kligman AM, Thorne EG, Topical therapy of actinic keratoses with tretinoin. In: Marks R (ed.). *Retinoids in cutaneous malignancy*. Blackwell Scientific Publications: Oxford, 1991, pp 66–73.
20. Moriarty M, Dunn J, Danagh A et al, Etretinate treatment in actinic keratoses. *Lancet* (1982) **i**: 364–5.
21. Berretti B, Grupper Ch, Cutaneous neoplasia and etretinate. In: Cunliffe WJ, Miller AJ (eds). *Retinoid therapy*, MTP Press: Lancaster, 1984, pp 195–9.
22. Marks R, Practical aspects of retinoid treatment for neoplastic disease of the skin. In: Marks R (ed.). *Retinoids in cutaneous malignancy*. Blackwell Scientific Publications: Oxford, 1991, ch 5.
23. Hughes BR, Marks R, Pearse AD, Clinical response and tissue effects of the treatment with retinoids of patients with solar keratoses and basal cell carcinomas. *J Am Acad Dermatol* (1988) **18**(3): 522–9.
24. Kingston T, Gaskell S, Marks R, The effects of a novel potent oral retinoid (RO13-6298) in the treatment of multiple solar keratoses and squamous cell epithelioma. *Eur J Cancer and Clin Oncol* (1983) **19**(9): 1201–5.
25. Shuttleworth D, Marks R, Griffin PJA et al, Treatment of cutaneous neoplasia with etretinate in renal transplant recipients. *Q J Med* (1988) **257**: 717–24.
26. Pearse AD, Gaskell S, Marks R, The effects of an aromatic retinoid (etretinate) on epidermal cell production and metabolism in normals and patients. *Br J Dermatol* (1986) **114**: 285–94.
27. Lippman SM, Meyskens FL Jr, Treatment of advanced squamous cell carcinoma of the skin with isotretinoin. *Ann Intern Med* (1987) **107**: 499–501.
28. Shalinsky DR, Bischoff ED, Gregory ML et al, Retinoid-induced suppression of squamous cell differentiation in human oral squamous cell carcinoma xenografts (line 1483) in athymic nude mice *Cancer Res* (1995) **55**: 3183–91.
29. Peck GL, Gross EG, Butkus D et al, Chemoprevention of basal cell carcinoma with isotretinoin. *J Am Acad Dermatol* (1982) **6**: 815–23.
30. Peck GL, DiGiovanna JJ, Sarnoff DS et al, Treatment and prevention of basal cell carcinoma with oral isotretinoin. *J Am Acad Dermatol* (1988) **19**(1/2): 176–85.
31. Goldberg LH, Hus SH, Alcalay J, Effectiveness of isotretinoin in preventing the appearance of basal cell carcinoma in basal cell naevus syndrome. *J Am Acad Dermatol* (1980) **21**: 144–5.
32. Tangrea JA, Edwards BK, Taylor PR et al, Long-term therapy with low-dose isotretinoin for prevention of basal cell carcinoma: a multicentre clinical trial. *J Natl Cancer Inst* (1992) **84**: 328–32.
33. Kraemer KH, DiGiovanna JJ, Moshell AB et al, Prevention of skin cancer in xeroderma pigmentosum with the use of oral isotretinoin. *N Engl J Med* (1988) **318**: 1633–7.
34. Schnitzler L, Retinïodes et prevention des epitheliomas cutanes, 1977–1987. *Ann Dermatol Vénéreol* (1987) **114**: 1537–43.
35. Bavinck JN, Tieben LM, Van der Woulde FJ et al, Prevention of skin cancer and reduction of keratotic skin lesions during acitretin therapy in renal transplant recipients: a double-blind, placebo-controlled study. *J Clin Oncol.* (1995) **13**: 1933–8.
36. Rook AH, Jaworsky C, Niguyen T et al, Beneficial effects of low-dose retinoid in combination with topical tretinoin for the

treatment and prophylaxis of premalignant and malignant skin lesions in renal transplant patients. *Transplantation* (1995) **59**: 14–19.
37. Jablonska S, Obalek S, Wolska H et al, Ro 10-9359 in epidermodysplasia verruciformis; preliminary report. In: Orfanos CE, Braun-Falco O, Farber EM et al (eds). *Retinoids: Advances in basic research and therapy*. Springer-Verlag: Berlin, 1981, pp 401–5.
38. Kanerva LO, Laurahanta J, Johansson E et al, Fine structure of epidermodysplasia verruciformis during long term etretinate treatment. *Dermatologica* (1984) **169**: 246–7.
39. Shuttleworth D, Marks R, Epidermal dysplasia and skeletal deformity in congenital poikiloderma (Rothman–Thompson syndrome). *Br J Dermatol* (1987) **117**: 377–84.
40. Alberts DS, Coulthard SW, Meyskens FL, Regression of aggressive laryngeal papillomatosis with isotretinoin. *J Biological Response Modifiers* (1986) **5**: 124–8.
41. Meyskens FL, Surwit ES, Clinical experience with topical tretinoin in the treatment of cervical dysplasia. *J Am Acad Dermatol* (1986) **15**: 826–9.
42. Cordero AA, Allevato MAJ, Barclay CA et al, Treatment of lichen planus and leukoplakia with oral retinoid Ro 10-9359. In: Orfanos CE, Braun-Falco O, Farber EM et al (eds). *Retinoids: Advances in basic research and therapy*. Springer-Verlag: Berlin, 1981, pp 273–8.
43. Stich HF, Rosin MP, Horby AP et al, Remission of oral leukoplakias and micro nuclei in tobacco/betel quid chewers treated with beta carotene and with beta carotene plus vitamin A. *Int J Cancer* (1988) **42**(2): 195–9.
44. Hong WK, Endicott J, Itri LM et al, 13-*cis*-retinoic acid in the treatment of oral leukoplakia. *N Engl J Med* (1986) **315**(24): 1501–5.
45. Gouveia J, Mathé G, Hercend T et al, Degree of bronchial metaplasia in heavy smokers and its regression after treatment with a retinoid. *Lancet*. (1982) **i**: 710–12.
46. Arnold AM, Browman GP, Levine MN et al, The effect of the synthetic cytology: results from a randomised trial. *Br J Cancer* (1992) **65**: 737–43.
47. Lotan R, Hendix MJC, Lippman SM, Retinoids in the management of melanoma. In: Marks R (ed.). *Retinoids in cutaneous malignancy*. Blackwell Scientific Publications: Oxford, 1991, pp 133–49.
48. Rustin GJS, Dische S, de Garis ST et al, Treatment of advanced malignant melanoma with interferon alpha and etretinate. *Eur J Cancer Clin Oncol* (1988) **24**: 783–4.
49. Claudy AL, Rouchouse B, Boucheron S et al, Treatment of cutaneous lymphoma with etretinate. *Br J Dermatol* (1983) **109**: 46–59.
50. Molin L, Thomsen K, Volden G et al, 13-*cis*-Retinoic acid in mycosis fungoides: a report from the Scandinavian Mycosis Fungoides Group. In: Saurat JH (ed.). *Retinoids: New trends in research and therapy*, Karger: Basel, 1985, pp 341–4.
51. Kessler JF, Jones SE, Levine N et al, Isotretinoin and cutaneous helper T-cell lymphoma (mycosis fungoides). *Arch Dermatol* (1987) **123**: 201–4.
52. Halpern AC, Schuchter LM, Elder DE et al, Effects of topical tretinoin on dysplastic nevi. *J Clin Oncol* (1994) **12**: 1028–35.

9 Photodamage

Ronald Marks

Introduction

In recent years there has been a growing appreciation that long-term exposure to sunlight carries significant health hazards as well as a few health benefits, and some undoubted subjective sensory pleasures. In particular it has been recognized that solar ultraviolet radiation (UVR) is capable of causing significant clinical damage to the skin. This fact has become of major importance in the past 50 years because social changes in this period have resulted in the increased exposure of affluent Westerners to ever more solar radiation,[1] and a frightening increase in skin cancer.

Increased vacation and leisure time, and the increased availability of relatively inexpensive air travel and all-in 'package' holidays to sunny resorts have put serious sun damage within the reach of almost everyone's pocket. The Mediterranean, the southern USA, the Caribbean, Mexico and more recently Thailand, Malaysia and East Africa have become the 'Meccas' of the sun-worshipping cult. This tendency has been compounded by other factors including an obsession of many to develop a deep and persistent sun-tan, and the development of sun-tan parlours with apparatus administering long-wave UVR to supply the incomprehensible and unnecessary demand.

A serious reduction in the protective ozone layer because of atmospheric pollution with long-lasting chlorofluorocarbons and nitrogen oxides is rapidly developing, and is threatening to aggravate the tendency to 'overdose' on UVR.[2] The increased exposure to solar UVR has resulted in an escalating incidence of both malignant melanoma and non-melanoma skin cancer which has been recorded in many centres.[3,4] This has provoked public health campaigns in Australia and the USA where death and disability from skin cancers have reached frightening proportions. Solar UVR also damages dermal connective tissue and other skin tissues to produce the clinical signs of what are incorrectly thought to be signs of aging and which has come to be known collectively as photoaging or dermatoheliosis. Neither term is entirely apposite, but the former is somewhat more euphonious and will be used here.

In addition to photocarcinogenesis and photoaging, chronic exposure to solar UVR results in immunological changes. The clinical consequences of these photoimmunological effects are less obvious than the other alterations but are none the less potentially very important.

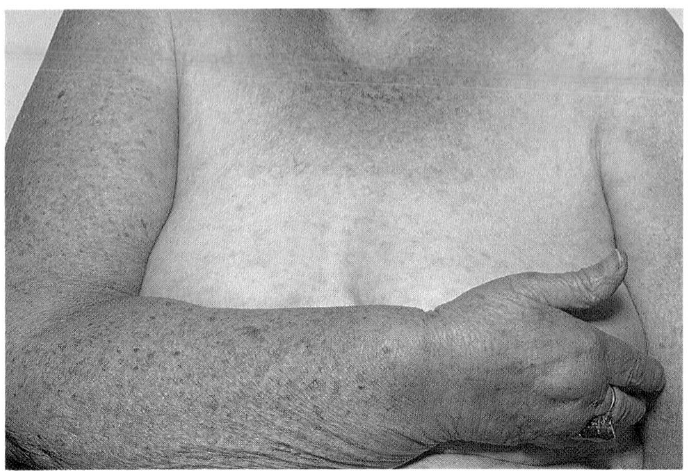

Figure 9.1

Exposed forearm skin and usually covered trunk skin demonstrating the alterations due to chronic solar exposure. The exposed skin shows mottled hyperpigmentation and irregular thickening.

Photoaging

Skin aging

Persistent exposure to the sun causes a distinctive cluster of signs that until recently were thought to be due to aging but are now recognized as predominantly the results of solar damage. All tissues and organs alter with the passing of the years but these changes of intrinsic aging are for the most part quite different from those due to solar exposure – which is why the term 'photoaging' is less than perfect. Contrast the difference in appearance of the forearm skin and the neighbouring truncal skin in Figure 9.1. The differences in texture and pigmentation are the result of solar damage and not the aging process itself, which is scarcely visible on the truncal skin.

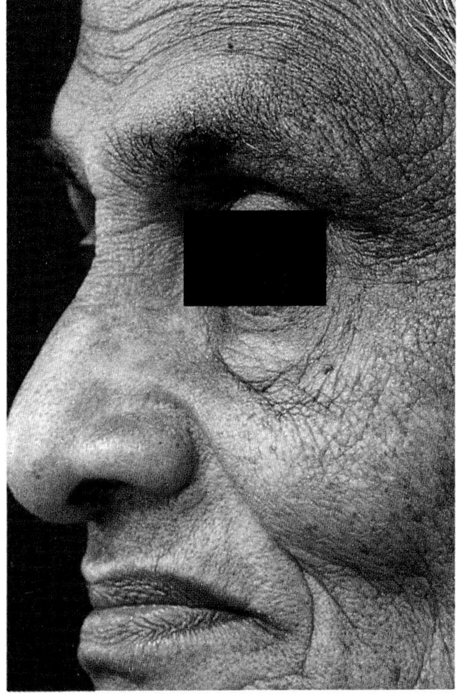

Figure 9.2

Hyperpigmentation due to solar damage in dark-skinned subject from Sri Lanka.

The influence of skin colour and racial type

Photodamage of all types is worse in fair-skinned individuals of skin types I and II without UVR protection from melanin. Those

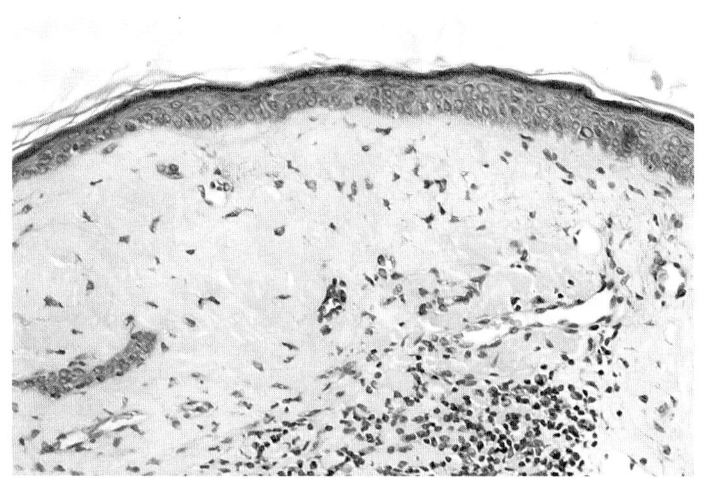

Figure 9.3

Histological section from area of chronic solar exposure to show solar elastotic degenerative change.

with light-blue eyes and a gingery complexion tend to sustain the most severe solar injury, but the most deeply pigmented individuals will also become photodamaged if the dose of UVR received is large enough. In some parts of Asia the quite darkly pigmented local population commonly manifest solar damage if they are habitually exposed to the sun but show more pigmentary anomalies than their Caucasian counterparts (Figure 9.2).

Some racial types, notably the Celtic populations originating from the British Isles, are peculiarly sensitive to solar injury. Whether this is entirely due to their usually quite fair skin or is due to some other inherent fault is uncertain. Some evidence is suggestive of an inherent metabolic fault.[5] Recent studies suggest that individuals of Celtic origin have a distinctive HLA profile with an excess of HLA-DR4, but the significance of this is not yet clear.

Solar elastosis

In sun-damaged skin the upper dermal collagenous connective tissue is replaced by a fragmented and disorganized material (Figure 9.3) which in places develops a homogeneous blob-like histological appearance. This altered connective tissue develops the staining reactions of elastin, even though it may not be identical with ordinary elastic tissue. This solar elastosis, as it is known, clearly imparts different mechanical properties to sun-damaged skin when compared with normal non-sun-damaged skin, accounting for the development of fine lines and wrinkles (Figure 9.4).[6] Not all facial wrinkles, lines, sags and furrows are due to solar damage, but the majority of fine lines, including those by the eyes, known as 'crow's feet', and those around the mouth, are the result of elastotic degenerative change. Odd white angulate and stellate scars are sometimes seen on the dorsa of forearms much damaged by the sun. The reasons for their appearance are not entirely clear.

Sun-damaged skin often has a sallow, yellowish tinge and it has been suggested that altered optical properties of the sun-damaged dermis may be responsible for this altered hue, although vascular and pigmentary alterations may contribute to it.

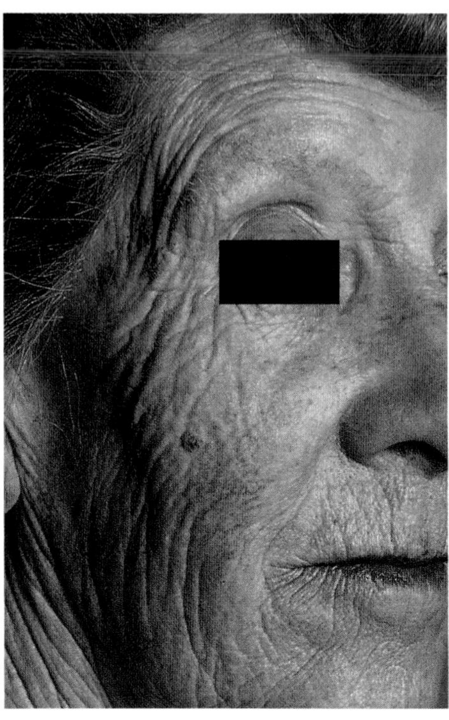

Figure 9.4

Fine lines and wrinkling on skin of face due to solar elastotic degenerative change.

Epidermal changes

Skin biopsies from exposed skin usually show irregular epidermal thickening as compared to thinning in intrinsically aged skin.[7] In addition, in severely photodamaged skin focal irregularities in cell and nuclear size, shape and staining reactions, as well as loss of cell polarity, may be seen (Figure 9.5). These changes of minimal dysplasia are especially pronounced in the areas around solar keratoses. The rate of cell proliferation, as judged by tritiated thymidine autoradiographic labelling indices, is increased in chronically sun-exposed skin.[8] These epidermal changes are probably responsible for the altered surface texture and apparent 'dryness' of chronically sun-exposed skin and are the precursors of neoplastic change (see later).

In non-exposed skin sites in the elderly there is a gradual reduction in number, size and activity of melanocytes, resulting in a gradual reduction in the degree of pigmentation of covered skin. This is not the case with sun-exposed skin. There is focal melanoyctic hyperplasia and overactivity[9] causing 'dyspigmentation' with hyperpigmented brown macules (one form of 'senile lentigo') as well as some general background increase in pigmentation (Figure 9.6).

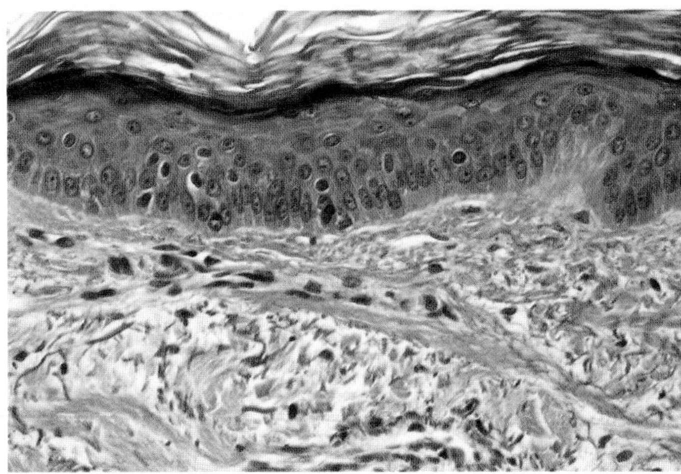

Figure 9.5

Histological section of chronically sun-exposed skin showing epidermal irregularities with heterogeneity in cell size and shape. The condition is known as minimal dysplasia.

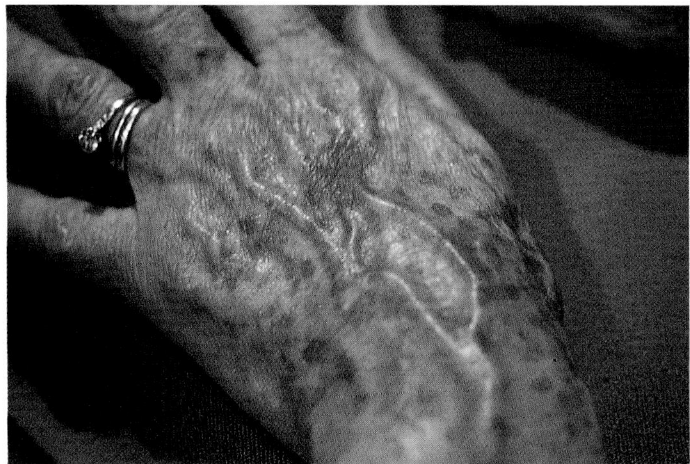

Figure 9.6

Senile lentigines and hyperpigmentation due to chronic solar exposure.

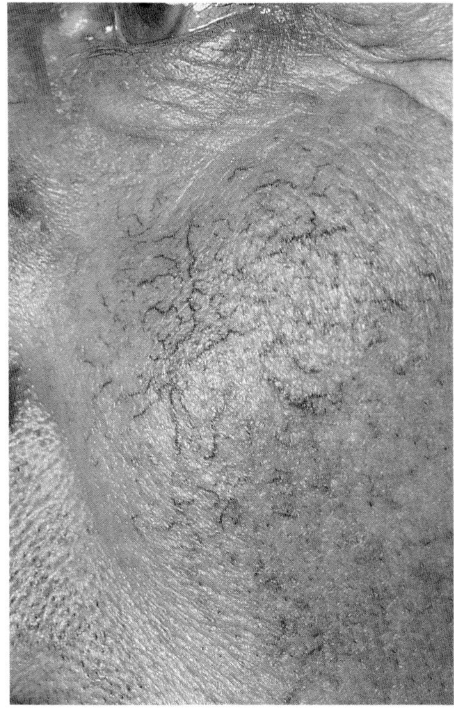

Figure 9.7

Telangiectasia in photodamaged skin.

The clinical lesion, known as senile lentigo, does not seem to represent a single entity. Solar keratoses, seborrhoeic warts and even lentigo maligna can all be clinically indistinguishable from senile lentigines. Some lesions even seem to be the result of a mixed pathological process.[10]

Langerhans cells are reduced in number in both light-exposed skin and covered skin.

Vascular and other alterations in photoaged skin

The superficial vasculature is gradually reduced in chronically sun-exposed skin.[11] Remaining vascular elements irregularly dilate, forming the telangiectatic network so often seen in photodamaged skin (Figure 9.7). The disorganized upper dermis fails in its function of giving support to the vessel walls, allowing the vessels to dilate passively. The 'English rose complexion' is largely a result of this vasodilatation rather than being a particular sign of health and vigour. The dilated and 'exposed' vasculature is more readily injured than in other sites, and this, together with photodamaged macrophages, accounts for the appearance and persistence of crimson bruises on the forearms known as senile purpura (probably better known as solar purpura).

Senile comedones have been thought to be a consequence of solar elastotic degenerative change and certainly in some cases there does seem to be marked elastosis at the site of these comedones. One study from the Cardiff group, however, failed to find a particular relationship of senile comedones with solar elastosis.[12] The comedones may be related to senile sebaceous gland hyperplasia, which also is probably not the result of solar elastosis.

The treatment of photoaging with topical retinoids

Studies with topical tretinoin

The use of topical tretinoin (all-*trans*-retinoic acid) to treat the signs of chronic solar damage was first described and subsequently popularized by Kligman in the mid-1980s. He observed alterations in the photodamaged facial skin of women receiving treatment with topical tretinoin for acne.[13] Kligman described a reduction in the fine lines around the eyes and mouth and improved skin colour with a decrease in the sallowness and the development of a rosy glow in the cheeks. At the same time there was a reduction in the telangiectatic vessels coursing over the photodamaged facial skin and a decrease in the numbers and prominence of senile lentigines. Together with these clinical benefits, Kligman found an increased epidermal thickness and in some cases the development of a 'repair band' of new dermal connective tissue pushing down the solar elastotic material.[14] These initial clinical observations were uncontrolled but well documented and supported by experimental work using the photodamaged hairless mouse model.[15] Further histological studies by Kligman demonstrated alterations in the stratum corneum in which the basket-weave pattern was supplanted by a thinner homogeneous structure. Epidermal cells in the thicker epidermis also seemed larger and 'healthier' than in photodamaged skin. Clinically photodamaged epidermis often shows minor dysplastic changes,[8] and in tretinoin-treated skin these undesirable alterations appear reduced. Tretinoin-treated skin also shows replacement of the sparse telangiectatic network by new dermal capillary blood vessels.[13]

These initial observations have been confirmed and extended by several clinical and experimental studies and the reader is referred to a review by Noble and Wagstaff.[16] More detailed investigation has revealed the deposition of mucin-like material in the epidermis of topical tretinoin-treated skin,[17] and provided evidence of the new dermal collagen synthesis in skin treated for prolonged periods.[18,19]

Controlled clinical trials

The initial clinical and histological observations were quickly supplemented by formal double-blind placebo-controlled clinical trials. The first of these was from Voorhees and his group in Ann Arbor, Michigan, and documented the result of a 4-month study of 0.1% tretinoin cream in 30 sun-damaged patients.[20] The tretinoin preparation and the vehicle were randomly assigned to either right or left forearm and the face was treated with the cream allotted to the left forearm. There was considerable improvement in the four clinical parameters assessed – fine wrinkling, coarse wrinkling, telangiectasia and roughness. There were also significant histological changes. There was marked epidermal thickening in tretinoin-treated skin compared with vehicle-treated skin (273 per cent). The stratum corneum from tretinoin-treated skin became compact and homogeneous in contrast to the usual basket-weave pattern observed. In addition to these alterations, a glycosaminoglycan-like material appeared in the stratum corneum of tretinoin-treated areas.

A further controlled clinical trial was performed by the Cardiff group.[21] A group of 20 photodamaged subjects were randomized to receive either 0.05% tretinoin or identical placebo material to one forearm and half-face while the other side received the alternative material. The study was conducted over a 12-week period with a follow-up at 16 weeks. Clinical assessments were made using visual analogue scales and, as well as biopsies, the non-invasive objective measurement method of pulsed A-scan ultrasound to determine skin thickness[22] was employed. Once again considerable improvement in the physical signs was noted on the tretinoin-treated sites. Both total skin thickness as determined by the ultrasound method and epidermal thickness assessed by histometric techniques were found to be increased. Neither of the above controlled studies detected any change in the profile of dermal connective tissue or solar elastosis. See further Table 8.1.

Large multicentre studies in the USA conducted by the Ortho Pharmaceutical Company, manufacturers of topical tretinoin, also produced incontrovertible evidence of marked clinical improvement in photodamaged skin.[23] Fine wrinkling, surface roughness and mottled hyperpigmentation were reduced by 0.05% tretinoin emollient cream. The effects were to some extent concentration dependent and also time dependent up to at least 6 months. Follow-up studies also seemed to indicate that after treatment stopped some of the improvement was lost, but as the life style of the treated individuals had also been altered it is difficult to be certain as to the reversibility or permanence of the clinical benefit induced. It did seem from these studies that improvement could be maintained after 1 year of topical treatment with the use of tretinoin emollient cream just once or three times weekly.

It has also become clear that, although the mottled dyspigmentation, fine lines and roughness are reduced, the more severe changes of deep wrinkles, skin laxness and very dark blemishes are not. Most patients treated are very appreciative of the improved appearance of the skin, and in particular are pleased with the 'bloom' and 'pinkness' of treated skin.

It is of interest to note that, in one study which compared the effects of 0.025%, 0.1% tretinoin preparations and vehicle, the two active creams were found to be equally effective clinically, although the more concentrated preparation had greater irritancy.[24]

Special techniques used to assess retinoid effects

These large-scale multicentre clinical studies have been supplemented by an objective technique that quantifies the degree of wrinkling lateral to the orbit (the so-called 'crow's foot' area) (Figure 9.8). The technique, known as optical profilometry, utilizes standardized skin surface replicas that are assessed by one centre using an image analysis device.[25] The data from these studies were presented as standardized roughness parameters in both the 'north–south' and the 'east–west' directions and demonstrated 'smoothing of the skin surface' at the sites examined.

Alterations in the relative amounts of dermal constituents of tretinoin-treated skin might be expected to be accompanied by

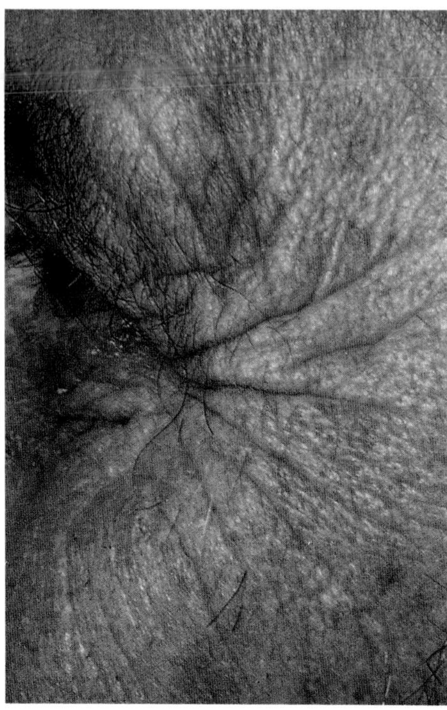

Figure 9.8

'Crow's feet' lines radiating from lateral edge of orbit.

changes in the mechanical properties of the areas treated. Although the Cardiff group recorded skin thickness increases in tretinoin–treated skin, no change was found in skin extensibility using a uniaxial extensometer. Curiously, changes in elasticity but not skin thickness were reported by Berardesca et al[26] but they employed a suction device to test the mechanical properties.

It seems likely that topical tretinoin does change the mechanical function of the skin but the detail of the alteration will depend on the state of the skin before treatment and duration of treatment, and its detection will depend on the test method used.

Effects on senile lentigines

A distressing feature of photodamage is dyspigmentation. Brown macules appearing over the backs of the hands and on the sides of the face cause a disproportionate amount of cosmetic discomfort. Their various names (e.g. age spots, liver spots, *médaillons de cimetière*) imply that their owners already have 'one foot in the grave'. They are a particular problem for Asian patients who dread the appearance of these lesions. The Voorhees group in Ann Arbour conducted a randomized, double-blind, vehicle-controlled trial of 0.1% tretinoin cream over a 10-month period. They found that the tretinoin preparation markedly lightened pigmented facial lesions (84 per cent of patients) compared with the vehicle-treated group (21 per cent). Gratifyingly, lesions that disappeared in the 10-month period did not reappear in the 6 months of follow-up.[27]

It is clear that, as Ortonne concludes in an excellent review, 'the effects of retinoic acid on pigment cells are multiple and complex'.[28] He further states, 'Although the beneficial action of topical tretinoin on pigmentary abnormalities of photoaged skin is well established, the basic mechanisms underlying the effects are not known'.

Effects of microcirculation

Many patients who have used topical tretinoin, as well as their physicians, have noted a 'rosy glow' of the cheeks after several weeks' treatment. For the most part this has been welcomed as a cosmetic benefit. As might be expected, this clinical feature is accompanied by the finding of increased skin capillary blood flow using a laser Doppler flow device.[29] Studies using an immunoradiometric assay for von Willebrand's factor antigen have also indicated an increased vascular endothelial cell mass in skin treated with topical tretinoin.[30]

Use of topical isotretinoin and other retinoids

The clinical benefits in patients with mild to moderate photodamage recorded with topical tretinoin have also been reported after the use of topical isotretinoin. In a double-blind, randomized, parallel-group multicentre study conducted by the Roche pharmaceutical company, 776 patients with mild to moderate photodamage were treated with either 0.05% isotretinoin cream for 12 weeks, followed by 0.1% isotretinoin cream for the next 24 weeks, or vehicle for 36 weeks.[31] Treatment with topical isotretinoin resulted in a statistically significant improvement in the overall appearance, the sallowness, the presence of senile lentigines and the skin surface texture. The improvements were evident with both patient and physician assessments.

One fascinating aspect of this study was a very carefully organized and meticulously performed assessment by a panel of five dermatologists of highly standardized photographs. The pre- and post-treatment photographic images could be projected on either of two screens, the allocation being randomized so that the assessors did not know which image was which. This ingenious technique also succeeded in demonstrating that the isotretinoin was superior to the vehicle in reducing the signs of photodamage.[32]

The successful trials of topical tretinoin and isotretinoin have stimulated searches for other topical retinoid drugs that could be effective in photodamage and have fewer adverse side-effects (see later). Retinyl palmitate has been shown to stimulate hairless mouse skin to produce epidermal thickening and an increased collagen content but has not yet been reported as an effective agent in humans. Retinyl palmitate (0.15 per cent) has been studied in a double-blind, randomized, vehicle-controlled clinical trial lasting 24 weeks in 80 subjects with photodamage. Disappointingly, no significant differences were found for either clinical signs or skin surface profilometric parameters. Retinol itself, in a topical formulation, has been claimed to have a therapeutic effect in photodamage. Other topical retinoids now licensed for the treatment of acne (Adapalene) and for psoriasis (tazarotene) will almost certainly be investigated for photodamage in the not too distant future.

Topical tretinoin and topical combinations for photodamaged dyspigmented skin

Numerous studies confirm the efficacy of topical tretinoin for photodamaged skin treatment.[13,23,33–38] Patients who have significant hyperpigmentation plus photodamaged skin may benefit from combinations of tretinoin with hydroquinone with or without low-potency topical corticorteroids. These combinations are derivatives of the original 'Kligman' formula and are often effective in treating hyperpigmentation (Figures 9.9 and 9.10). It is essential that anyone being treated for photodamage should be encouraged to apply sunscreens each morning.

Adverse side-effects

A drawback of the use of these topical retinoids has been their tendency to irritate the skin. Treated areas tend to become pink, slightly scaly, and sore or pruritic. This 'retinoid dermatitis' is to some extent concentration dependent. It becomes less prevalent and less troublesome during treatment in the months that follow and is rarely the reason for a patient stopping treatment. Fair-skinned blue-eyed subjects seem more vulnerable than darker-skinned individuals.

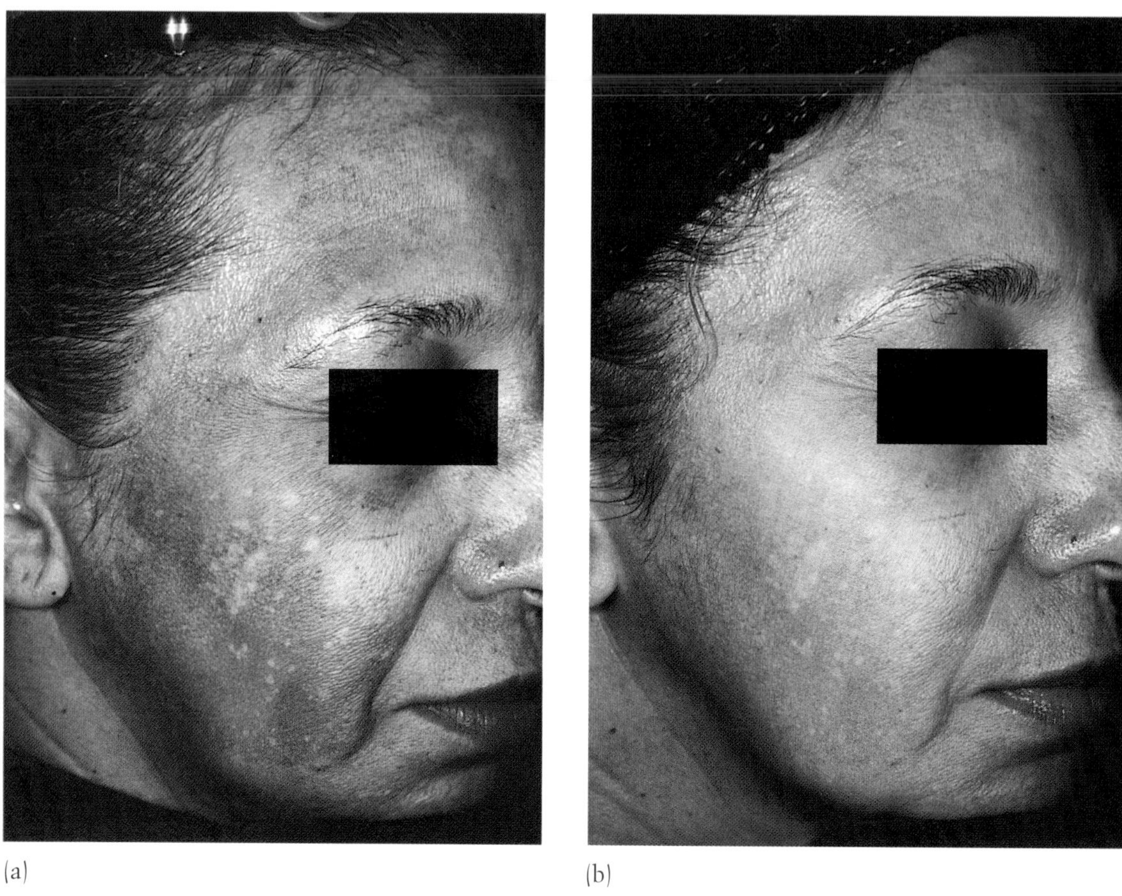

(a) (b)

Figure 9.9

(a) Photodamaged skin with severe melanosis; **(b)** patient in **(a)** following 12 weeks' therapy with tretinoin 0.05%, hydroquinone 5%, Desonide 0.01% cream nightly. (Courtesy of NJ Lowe, MD.)

However, as a study of 0.1% tretinoin cream in melasma in black-skinned patients showed,[34] even deeply pigmented individuals can be successfully treated.[39] In one study only 5 per cent of patients treated with topical 0.05% isotretinoin developed 'severe tolerability reactions'[32] but as the system of assessment was different from that employed in studies using topical tretinoin it is not clear whether the two isomers are equally irritant or not. In any event, most such reactions can be improved by liberal use of emollients or, if required, weak topical corticosteroids. A reduced frequency of application (for example, once every 2 or even 3 days) will also improve the irritation. All patients should be warned of the possibility of irritation after the use of topical retinoids and urged to use the preparation less frequently rather than to stop treatment.

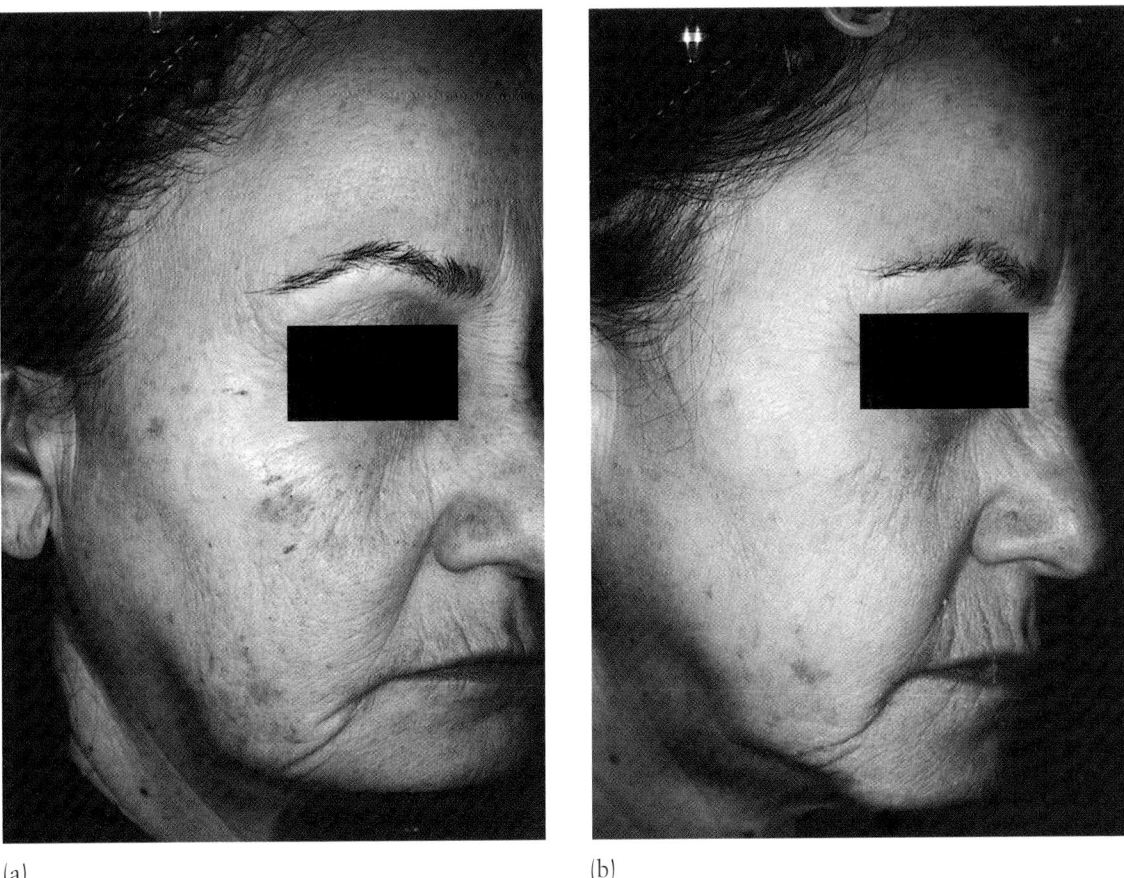

(a) (b)

Figure 9.10

(a) Photodamaged skin with solar lentigo; **(b)** patient in **(a)** after treatment for 12 weeks with tretinoin 0.05%, hydroquinone 5%, and Desonide 0.01% cream nightly. (Courtesy of NJ Lowe, MD.)

The possibility of more serious adverse side-effects has often been discussed but not substantiated. Experiments in mice have indicated that topical tretinoin can in some instances promote UVR-induced skin cancer and in other cases can inhibit the development of UVR-induced neoplasia, but yet other experiments have shown no effect on skin cancer formation of any kind attributable to tretinoin. No epidemiological or clinical evidence in humans has been reported that could incriminate topical tretinoin in this regard. Indeed topical tretinoin has been used as a treatment for solar keratoses (see chapter 8).

The other major concern has been the possibility of teratogenicity from the absorption of tretinoin through the skin. Percutaneous penetration of topical tretinoin occurs to a limited degree only – less than 5 per cent of an applied dose over a 24-h period. In addition, experiments have shown that it is very difficult to raise the blood levels of tretinoin above normal by application of tretinoin to large areas of skin. A recent report describes a study in which 230 women who had used tretinoin topically in the first trimester of pregnancy were compared with 430 age-matched women who had not used any preparation containing tretinoin during their pregnancy. There was no increase in the prevalence of major anomalies among babies born to the tretinoin-exposed women, and indeed the overall prevalence rate in this group was 1.9 per cent compared with 2.9 per cent in the control group.[40] Thus despite fears, there has been no evidence of a teratogenic effect from the use of topical tretinoin.

Mode of action

The mode of action of topical retinoids in photodamage is unclear. The epidermal stimulation and the reduction in melanin synthesis caused by topical retinoids may partially explain the therapeutic benefit experienced, but it is quite clear this is not the entire story. When hairless mice are irradiated with UVR a band of solar elastotic degenerative change develops below the epidermis, just as in humans. When such mice are treated by either topical tretinoin or topical isotretinoin new dermal connective tissue is formed above the abnormal elastotic tissue, so that a repair zone is found.[41] This process has rarely been identified in human skin treated with topical retinoids and presumably the reason for this is the different periods of time over which humans and mice have been treated when compared with the expected life span of the two species. Increase in thickness in the normal dermal collagen in the subepidermal zone in the skin of photodamaged subjects treated for a mean of 25 months with 0.05% tretinoin was detected in 11 patients.[42] However, further studies are needed to confirm this observation. After treatment with tretinoin, new anchoring fibrils beneath the basal lamina have been detected ultrastructurally and it is certainly the case that there is an increase of mucosubstances throughout the skin after topical retinoid treatment. It would seem likely that a substantial proportion of the therapeutic effect is due to the stimulation of dermal fibroblasts and the increased rate of synthesis of all components of the dermal extracellular matrix.

Some physicians have remained unconvinced of the efficacy of topical retinoids in chronic photodamage and have suggested that any apparent clinical benefit stems from the irritating effects of these compounds and the resulting oedema of the skin that they cause. It is certainly the case that transient improvements in the appearance of photodamage can be produced by agents such as emollients that increase skin hydration, but these changes last for hours only and affect only one component of the photodamaged appearance – that is, the fine lines. It is of interest to note that in all the multicentre controlled studies a degree of benefit has been noted in the control vehicle only (placebo) group. Often this benefit has been sufficient to suggest that it may be clinically relevant in some subjects, that is, they may have looked somewhat less photodamaged. The basis of this unexpected improvement in placebo-treated subjects is mysterious. One explanation may be that the sun-avoidance regimen which the subjects followed may have allowed sufficient repair to have occurred without further damage – the net result being clinical improvement. It is also possible that the act of application of a topical agent itself may have mechanically stimulated the repair processes. In this respect it is worthwhile noting that in a study comparing the effects of 0.05% tretinoin with a cream containing an abrasive on objective parameters of skin structure and function, the abrasive preparation was found to be at least as 'stimulating' as the tretinoin.[43] Irritating sodium lauryl sulphate solutions were also found to alter biochemical pathways significantly in skin in a similar manner to tretinoin.[44]

An explanation for these curious results and anomalous observations could be that some of the clinical effects observed with topical tretinoin are receptor mediated and some are dependent on various other mechanisms.

APPENDIX

Selection of concentration

For treatment of photodamaged facial skin

Treatment may be initiated for most patients with tretinoin 0.025% or 0.05% cream. In patients with skin types I and II, concentrations above this lead to erythema and desquamation. This is frequently more pronounced in dry, low-humid times of year, i.e. the winter months in northern Europe and the USA. During this time of the year it is necessary to reduce the concentration and/or frequency of the tretinoin.

Greater patient tolerance may often be established by initiating at the lowest (0.025%) tretinoin cream concentration and increasing the concentration after 2 or 4 weeks of therapy to 0.05% cream. If the patient tolerates this concentration he or she may benefit from treatment with 0.1% cream.

Forearm and dorsal hand skin

The concentration selected for the treatment of photodamaged forearm and dorsal hand skin can be higher than that for the face. Patients will frequently tolerate 0.1% tretinoin cream on the forearms and dorsal hands. Some patients will actually tolerate tretinoin gel 0.01% and 0.015%. Adequate moisturization is also needed with the gel.

A sensible routine is for a careful morning application of a moisturizing sunscreen of at least Sun Protection Factor 15 to the skin areas exposed to the sun. The patient may apply a moisturizer in the early evening. The tretinoin is applied last thing at night, allowing approximately 30 minutes before bedtime to allow the preparation to be percutaneously absorbed.

Advice given to patients

An example of the information given to the patient by NJ Lowe is as follows.

How to use tretinoin cream

To get the best results from tretinoin cream therapy, it is necessary to use it properly.

Forget about the instructions given for other products and the advice of friends. Just stick to the special plan your physician has laid out for you and be patient. Remember, when tretinoin cream is used properly, many users see improvement by 12 weeks. Again, FOLLOW INSTRUCTIONS; BE PATIENT; DON'T START AND STOP THERAPY ON YOUR OWN; IF YOU HAVE ANY QUESTIONS, ASK YOUR PHYSICIAN.

To help you use the medication correctly, keep these simple instructions in mind.

- Apply TRETINOIN CREAM once daily before bedtime or as directed by your physician. First wash with a mild soap and dry your skin gently.
- It is better not to use more than the amount suggested by your physician or to apply more frequently than instructed. Too much may irritate your skin, waste medicament and won't give faster results.
- Keep the medication away from the corners of the nose, mouth, eyes and open wounds. Spread away from these areas when applying.
- Squeeze about a half-inch or less of cream onto the fingertip. While that should be enough for your whole face, you may find that you need slightly less to do the job after you have some experience with the medication. The medication should become invisible almost immediately. If it is still visible, you are using too much. Cover the affected area lightly with cream by first dabbing it in your forehead, chin and both cheeks, then spreading it over the entire affected area. Smooth gently into the skin.
- SUNSCREENS: a sunscreen with Sun Protection Factor of 15 or greater must be used each morning.
- MOISTURIZER: a non-acnegenic moisturizer may be used twice daily.

What to expect with your new treatment

There may be some discomfort during the early days of treatment. Some patients also notice that their skin begins to take on a blush.

These reactions do not happen to everyone. If they do, it is just your skin adjusting to tretinoin cream and this usually subsides within 2–4 weeks. These reactions can usually be minimized by following instructions carefully. Should the effects become excessively troublesome, consult your physician.

References

1. Marks R, *The sun and your skin.* Macdonald Optima: London, 1988.
2. Russell Rones R, Ozone depletion and its effects on human populations. *Br J Dermatol* (1922) **127** (suppl 41): 2–6.
3. McHenry PM, Hole DJ, MacKie RM, Melanoma in people aged 65 and over in Scotland, 1979–89. *Br Med J* (1993) **304**: 756–9.
4. Harvey I, Frankel SJ, Shalom D et al, Non melanoma skin cancer: Questions concerning its distribution and natural history. *Br Med J* (1989) **299**: 1118–20.
5. Abo-Darub JM, Mackie R, Pitts JD, DNA repair in cells from patients with actinic keratosis. *J Invest Dermatol* (1983) **80**: 214–44.
6. Matsuoka LY, Uitto J, Alterations in the elastic fibres in cutaneous aging and solar elastosis. In: AK Balin, AM Kligman (eds). *Aging and the skin.* Raven Press: New York, 1989, ch 7.
7. Marks R, Berth-Jones J, Black DR et al, The effects of photoaging and intrinsic aging on epidermal structure and function. *Giornale Italiano di Chirurgia Dermatologica ed Oncologia* (1987) **2**(3–4): 252–63.
8. Pearse AD, Marks R, Actinic keratoses and the epidermis on which they arise. *Br J Dermatol* (1977) **96**: 45–50.

9. Gilchrest BA, Blog FB, Szabo G, Effects of ageing and chronic sun exposure on melanocytes in human skin. *J Invest Dermatol* (1979) **73**: 77–83.
10. Lever LR, Marks R, Pigmented facial macules: a sign of photoaging? In: Marks R, Plewig G (eds). *The environmental threat to the skin.* Martin Dunitz: London, 1992, pp 91–6.
11. Braverman IM, Elastic fiber and microvascular abnormalities in aging skin. In: AM Kligman, Y Takase (eds). *Cutaneous aging.* University of Tokyo Press, 1988, p 369.
12. Kumar R, Marks R, Sebaceous gland hyperplasia and senile comedones: a prevalence study in elderly hospitalized patients. *Br J Dermatol* (1987) **117**: 231–6.
13. Kligman AM, Grove GL, Hirose R et al, Topical tretinoin for photoaged skin. *J Am Acad Dermatol* (1986) **15**: 836–59.
14. Kligman AM, Graham GF, Histological changes in facial skin after daily application of tretinoin for 5 to 6 years. *J Dermatol Treat* (1993) **4**: 113–17.
15. Kligman LH, Effects of all trans retinoic acid on the dermis of hairless mice. *J Am Acad Dermatol* (1986) **15**: 779–85.
16. Noble S, Wagstaff AJ, Tretinoin: A review of its pharmacological properties and clinical efficacy in the treatment of photodamaged skin. *Drugs Aging* (1995) **6**: 479–96.
17. Bhawan J, Gonzalez-Serva A, Nehal K et al, Effects of tretinoin on photodamaged skin. A histologic study. *Arch Dermatol* (1991) **127**: 666–72.
18. Marks R, The pathology of chronic solar damage and the effects of topical tretinoin. *J Dermatol Treat* (1996) **7** (suppl 2): S13–17.
19. Griffiths CEM, Russman AN, Mayumdar G et al, Restoration of collagen formation in photodamaged skin by tretinoin (retinoic acid). *N Engl J Med* (1993) **329**: 530–5.
20. Weiss JS, Ellis CN, Headington JT et al, Treatment of photodamaged facial skin with topical tretinoin. *J Am Med Assoc* (1988) **259**: 527–32.
21. Lever L, Kumar P, Marks R, Topical retinoic acid in the treatment of solar elastotic degeneration. *Br J Dermatol* (1990) **122**: 91–8.
22. Tan CY, Statham B, Marks R et al, Skin thickness measurement by pulsed ultrasound: its reproducibility, validation and variability. *Br J Dermatol* (1982) **106**: 657–67.
23. Olsen EA, Katz I, Levine N et al, Tretinoin emollient cream: a new therapy for photodamaged skin. *J Am Acad Dermatol* (1992) **26**: 215–24.
24. Griffiths CEM, Kang S, Ellis CN et al, Two concentrations of topical tretinoin (retinoic acid) cause similar improvement of photoaging, but different degrees of irritation. *Arch Dermatol* (1995) **131**: 1037–44.
25. Grove GL, Grove MJ, Leyden JJ, Optical profilometry: an objective method for the quantification of facial wrinkles. *J Am Acad Dermatol* (1989) **21**: 631–7.
26. Berardesca E, Gabba P, Farinelli N et al, In vivo tretinoin-induced changes in skin mechanical properties. *Br J Dermatol* (1990) **122**: 525–9.
27. Rafal ES, Griffiths CEM, Ditre CM et al, Topical tretinoin (retinoid acid) treatment for liver spots associated with photodamage. *N Engl J Med* (1992) **326**: 368–74.
28. Ortonne J-P, Retinoic acid and pigment cells: a review of in-vitro and in-vivo studies. *Br J Dermatol* (1992) **127** (suppl 41): 43–7.
29. Marks R, Edwards C, The measurement of photodamage. *Br J Dermatol* (1992) **127** (suppl 41): 7–13.
30. Mourad MM, Marks R, Giddings G, Effects of retinoic acid and corticosteroids on capillary endothelium of human skin (Abstract). *J Invest Dermatol* (1989) **92**: 393.
31. Sendagorta E, Lesiewicz J, Armstrong RB, Toptical isotretinoin for photodamaged skin. *J Am Acad Dermatol* (1992) **27**(6): S15–18.
32. Epstein J, Photocarcinogenesis and topical retinoids. In: R Marks (ed.). *Retinoids in cutaneous malignancy.* Blackwell Scientific Publications: Oxford, 1991, pp 171–82.
33. Leyden JJ, Tretinoin therapy in photoageing: historical perspective. *Br J Dermatol* (1990) **122** (suppl 35): 83–6.
34. Leyden JJ, Grove GL, Grove MJ et al, Treatment of photodamaged facial skin with topical tretinoin. *J Am Acad Dermatol* (1989) **21**: 638–44.
35. Ellis CN, Weiss JS, Hamilton TA et al, Sustained improvement with prolonged topical tretinoin (retinoic acid) for photoaged skin. *J Am Acad Dermatol* (1990) **23**: 629–37.
36. Weinstein GD, Nigra TP, Pochi PE et al, Topical tretinoin for treatment of photodamaged skin: a

multicenter study. *Arch Dermatol* (1991) **127**: 659–65.

37. Grove GL, Grove MJ, Leyden JJ et al, Skin replica analysis of photodamaged skin after therapy with tretinoin emollient cream. *J Am Acad Dermatol* (1991) **25**: 231–7.
38. Thorne EG, Long-term clinical experience with a topical retinoid. *Br J Dermatol* (1992) **127** (suppl. 41): 31–6.
39. Kimbraugh-Green CK, Griffiths CEM, Finkel LJ et al, Topical retinoic acid (Tretinoin) for melasma in black patients. *Arch Dermatol* (1994) **130**: 727–33.
40. Jick SS, Terris BZ, Jick H, First trimester topical tretinoin and congenital disorders. *Lancet* (1993) **341**: 1181–2.
41. Kligman LH, Duo CH, Kligman AM, Topical retinoic acid enhances the repair of ultraviolet-damaged dermal connective tissue. *Connective Tissue Res* (1994) **12**: 139–50.
42. Marks R, The pathology of chronic solar damage and the effects of topical tretinoin. *J Dermatol Treat* (1996) **7** (suppl 2): 513–17.
43. Marks R, Hill S, Barton SP, The effects of an abrasive agent on normal skin and on photoaged skin in comparison with topical tretinoin. *Br J Dermatol* (1990) **123**: 457–66.
44. Griffiths CEM, Finkel LJ, Tranfaglia MG et al, An in vivo experimental model for effects of topical retinoic acid in human skin. *Br J Dermatol* (1988) **129**: 389–94.

10 Keratinization disorders

Nicholas J Lowe

Introduction

Systemic retinoids have revolutionized the management of patients with severe keratinizing disorders. These diseases are all characterized by abnormal epidermal differentiation with varying degrees of cutaneous inflammation. In the case of Darier's disease there is also acantholysis.

Prior to the availability of systemic retinoids there was little that the clinician could offer patients with these disorders, with the exception of topical emollients, retinoic acid and keratolytic agents. In the case of pityriasis ruba pilaris (PRP) there are other therapeutic options which will be discussed later in this chapter.

When treating patients with these disorders, with the exception of acute adult-onset PRP (usually a self-limiting disease), the physician must remember that these diseases are chronic, usually life-long disorders. Because of this fact the chronic use of systemic retinoids with their known toxicity problems has to be considered very carefully. Several different systemic retinoids have been shown to be effective in improving these diseases. They include isotretinoin, etretinate and acitretin. This chapter deals with each of these keratinizing disorders in detail.

Lamellar ichthyosis (non-bullous ichthyosiform erythroderma)

There are at least two forms of lamellar ichthyosis recently identified following studies showing variations of the disease characterized by different degrees of inflammation. The disease may start at or shortly after birth, with some children showing the first evidence of disease as a collodion baby. Both forms of the disease are manifested by large areas of plate-like hyperkeratosis covering most parts of the skin. The inflammatory form of lamellar ichthyosis is characterized by more severe erythema in addition to abnormal scale accumulation, and a tendency for more involvement of the face. The two forms of the disease may have different modes of inheritance.

Both forms of the disease usually respond well to the different systemic retinoids. Women of childbearing potential are best treated with isotretinoin or acitretin. However, males and non-fertile women may be treated with etretinate. There is usually increased desquamation and subsequent decreased thickness of scale in these patients treated with systemic retinoids.

Table 10.1 Suggested doses of systemic retinoids in disorders of keratinization

	Isotretinoin	*Etretinate*	*Acitretin*
Starting dose (mg/kg per day)	1–2	0.75–1.5	0.5–1
Maintenance dose (mg/kg per day)	0.5–1	0.5–1	0.25–0.75

Suggested starting doses and maintenance doses for these three retinoids are given in Table 10.1.

Complications include mucocutaneous toxicity and increased skin fragility. Skin infections may occur particularly in the skin folds and perioral area. Desquamation of the palms and soles can lead to tenderness of the skin which may become disabling. Drug-induced alopecia is also seen in approximately 20–25 per cent of patients. The general considerations of systemic retinoid toxicity are reviewed in chapter 12. Of particular concern with these patients is the long-term use of systemic retinoids and the possibility of skeletal hyperostosis.

Epidermolytic hyperkeratosis (bullous ichthyosiform erythroderma)

This is a severely disfiguring and disabling disease that may be improved with systemic retinoids (Figures 10.1–10.5). It is usually an autosomal dominantly inherited disease, although in many patients it occurs as an apparently spontaneous mutation. Clinical signs are severe generalized hyperkeratosis with relatively little inflammation, and a characteristic 'picket fence' hyperkeratosis usually seen in the flexural skin sites. Skin infections such as impetigo occur and skin stiffness and lack of mobility are frequently seen in these patients.

As with lamellar ichthyosis the availability of systemic retinoids has provided a treatment option for patients with epidermolytic hyperkeratosis where none previously existed. Because it is a persistent disease patients need to be aware that the drug will have to be used long term and the disease will relapse on discontinuation of therapy. Another problem associated with systemic retinoids is an increase in skin fragility because of increased superficial desquamation of the hyperkeratosis. Some patients develop bullous lesions and impetigo on retinoid therapy for this disease.

X-linked recessive ichthyosis

X-linked recessive ichthyosis is usually too mild to be treated with systemic retinoids.

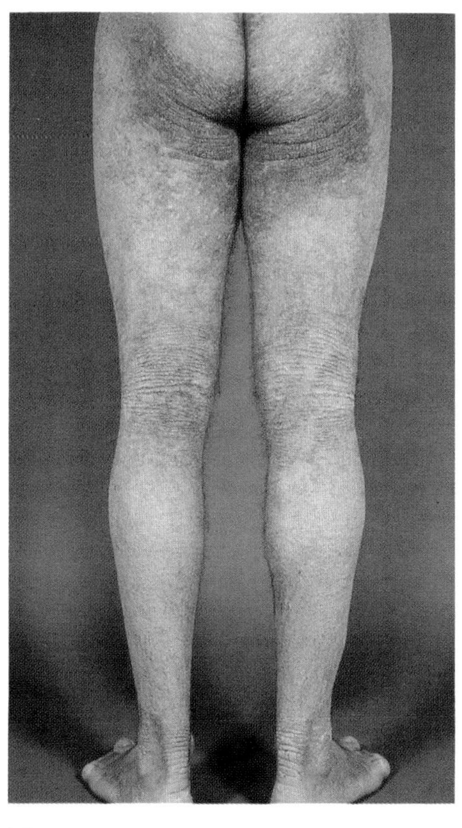

(a)

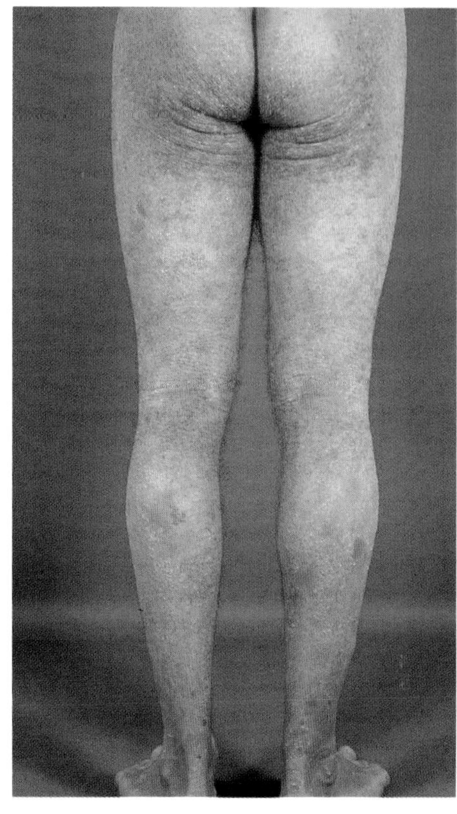

(b)

Figure 10.1

(a) Patient with epidermolytic hyperkeratosis before treatment with etretinate 0.75 mg/kg per day. **(b)** The same patient after treatment.

Because some patients experience significant disfigurement from the disease, some cases have been treated with acitretin using doses of 35 mg/day, with a marked improvement or total clearing. An adequate maintenance dose may be 10 mg/day.

Harlequin fetus syndrome

Harlequin fetus syndrome is a severe neonatal skin disorder. A striking improvement may be seen after etretinate therapy in this skin condition, which may be fatal if

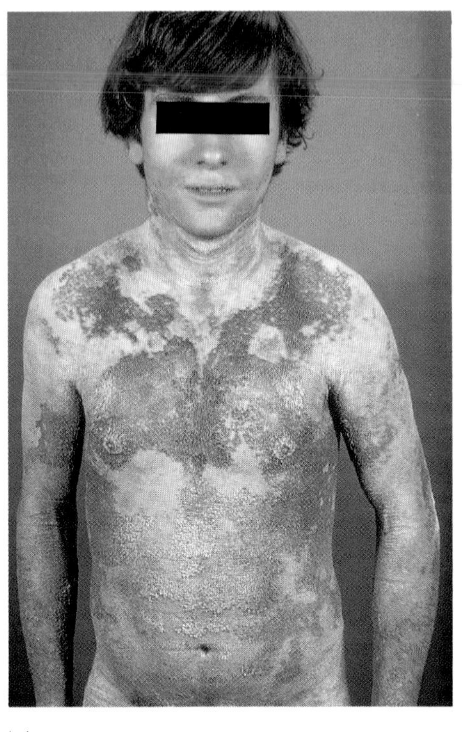

(a)

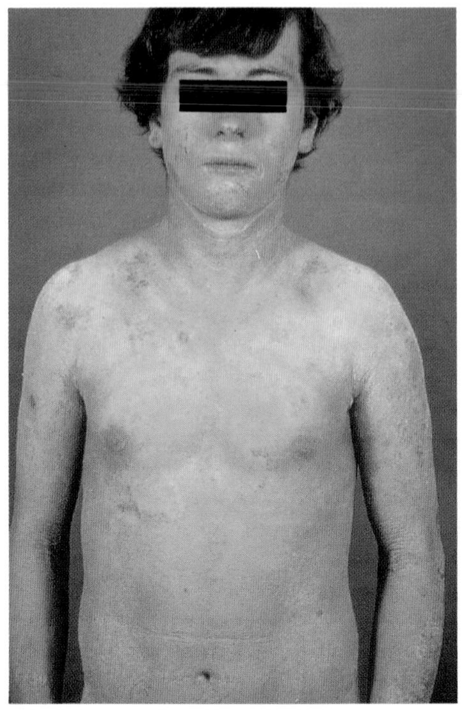

(b)

Figure 10.2

(a) Same patient as in Figure 10.1 before treatment. **(b)** The same patient after treatment.

untreated. It has been reported that there is no relapse after discontinuation of etretinate in some treated patients. Others have reported a rapid improvement in Harlequin fetus syndrome with acitretin at a dose of 1 mg/kg per day.

Erythrokeratodermia variabilis

Erythrokeratodermia variabilis (Mendes da Costa disease) is an autosomal dominant disorder of keratinization characterized by varying configurations of sharply demarcated

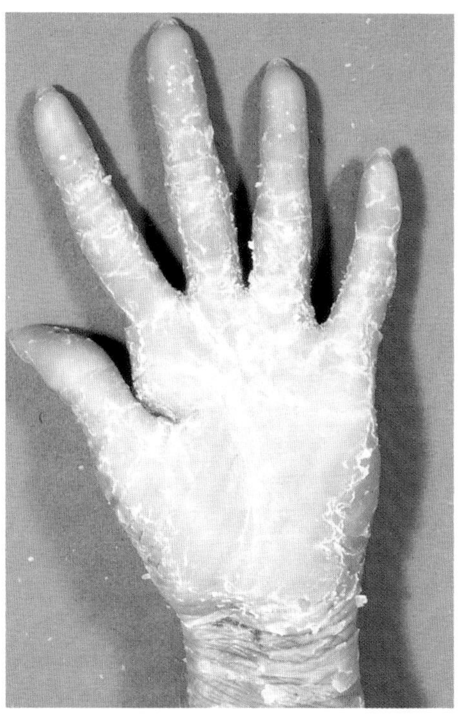

(a)

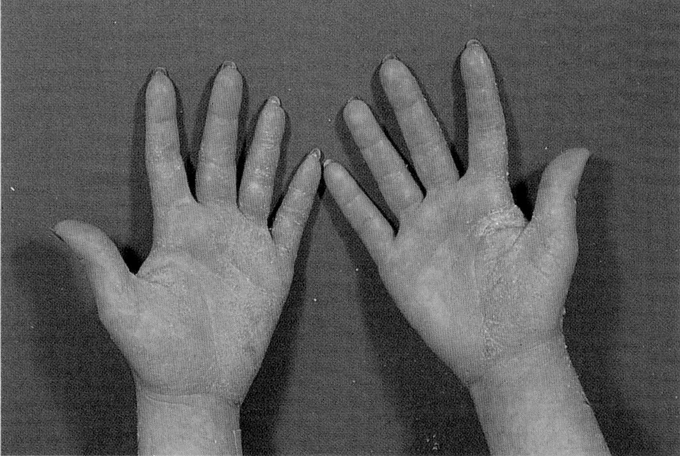

(b)

Figure 10.3

(**a**) Palmar keratoderma in epidermolytic hyperkeratosis before treatment with etretinate 0.75 mg/kg per day.
(**b**) The same patient after treatment.

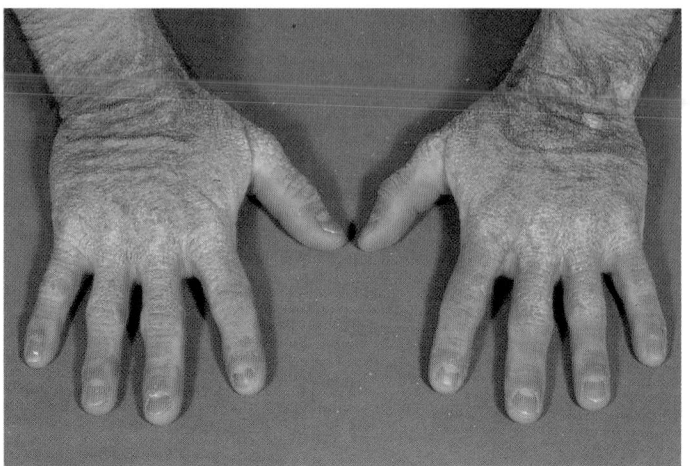

(a)

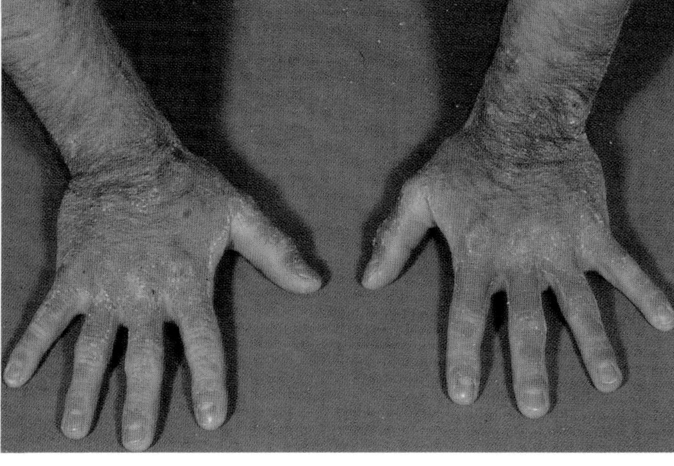

(b)

Figure 10.4

(a) Epidermolytic hyperkeratosis before treatment with etretinate 1 mg/kg per day for 3 months.
(b) The same patient after treatment.

erythematous hyperkeratotic plaques. Good results have been reported with etretinate.

Darier's disease

Darier's disease is an important indication for systemic retinoid therapy. Etretinate results in excellent improvement using doses between 0.25 and 0.75 mg/kg per day. Acitretin 10–30 mg/day has also been reported to produce an impressive improvement. It is advisable to commence treatment with relatively low doses of acitretin 10–25 mg/day, adjusting the dose gradually in the light of the narrow therapeutic margin and large interindividual variability in dose–response relationship. In fertile female patients isotretinoin is effective at doses between 0.5 and 1 mg/kg per day, and may be used where acitretin is not

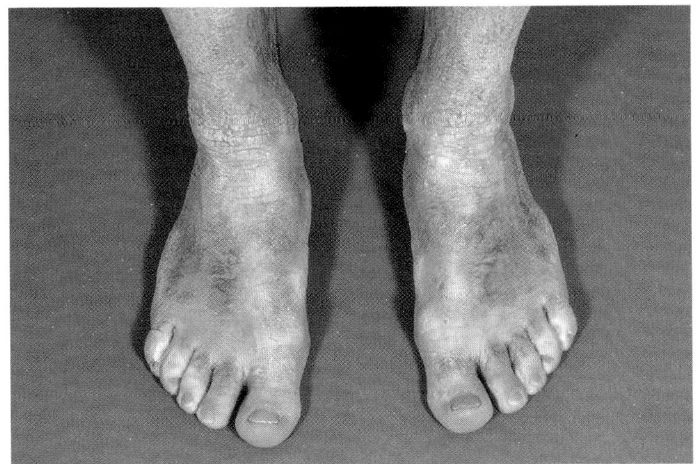

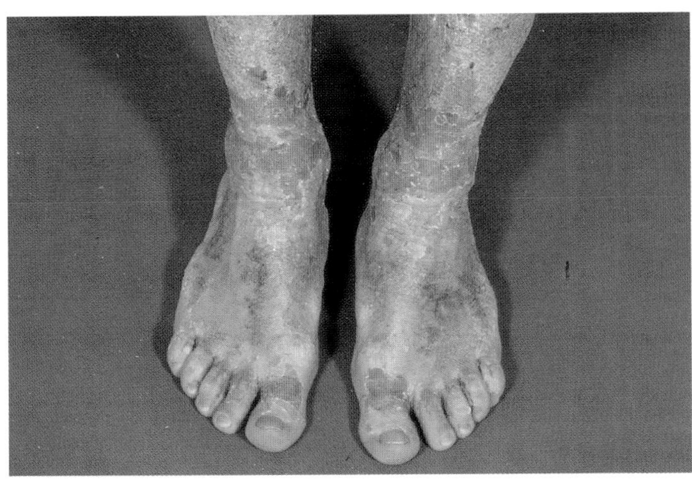

(b)

Figure 10.5

(a) Bullous ichthyosiform erythroderma (epidermolytic hyperkeratosis). **(b)** The same patient on treatment with etretinate 75 mg/day.

yet available, for example in the USA (see Figures 10.6 and 10.7).

Hereditary palmoplantar keratodermas

Before a systemic retinoid is prescribed for a patient with palmoplantar keratoderma, it is wise to establish a precise diagnosis based on the clinical observations and histology. In particular, it is of importance to avoid the use of retinoids in palmoplantar keratoderma of the epidermolytic type, as painful erosions may cause the patient's condition to deteriorate. Cautious low doses of the systemic retinoids isotretinoin, etretinate or acitretin and frequent clinical evaluation are advised. Acitretin has been prescribed in patients with Papillon–Levèvre syndrome with excellent

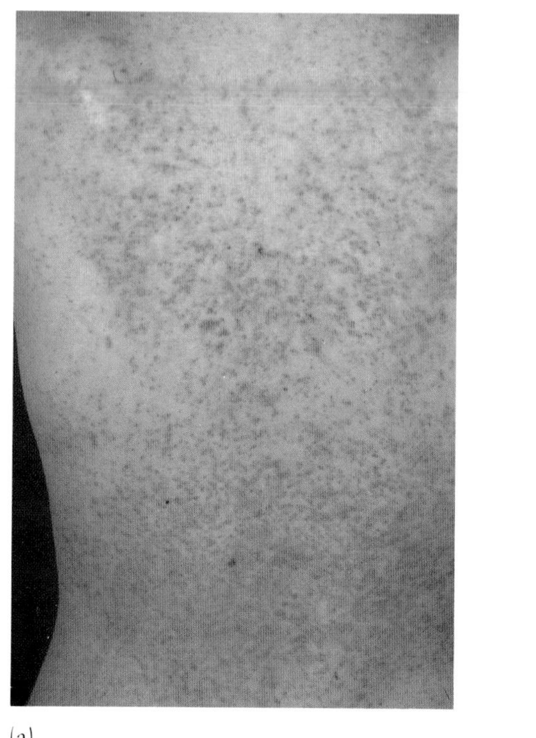

(a)

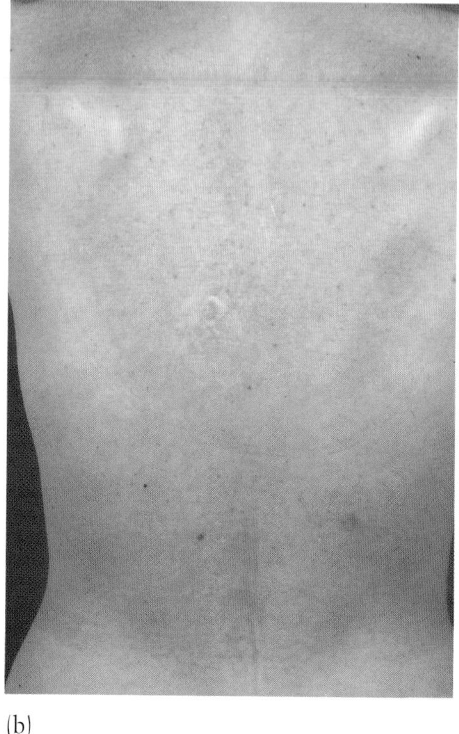

(b)

Figure 10.6

(a) Darier's disease before treatment with isotretinoin 1 mg/kg per day. **(b)** The same patient after treatment.

results, and it is suggested that early treatment may result in restoration of normal definition in some patients with this syndrome.

Pityriasis rubra pilaris

There have been a number of case reports of PRP patients successfully treated with etretinate. Kanerva et al[1] reported an 80 per cent response rate, while Marks et al[2] found a 67 per cent response rate. Borok and Lowe[3] reviewed a group of 18 patients seen between 1978 and 1987 and found that etretinate-treated patients resolved at lower doses and also clearly slightly faster than isotretinoin-treated patients, 5 months versus 6.5 months, respectively. Adult-onset PRP in retinoid-treated patients resolves significantly faster than that in untreated patients. In further

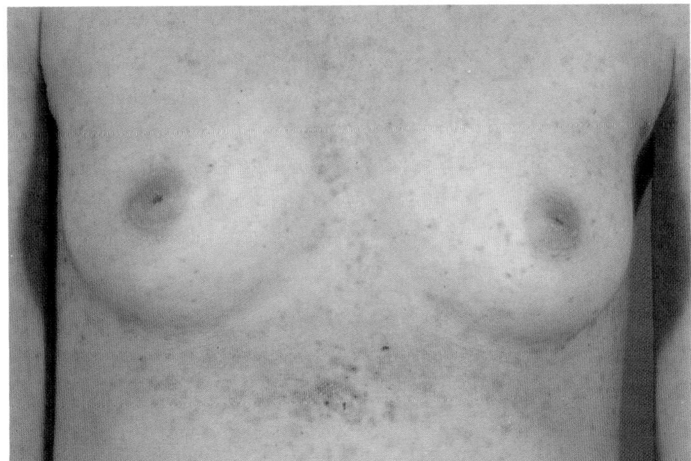

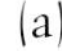

(a)

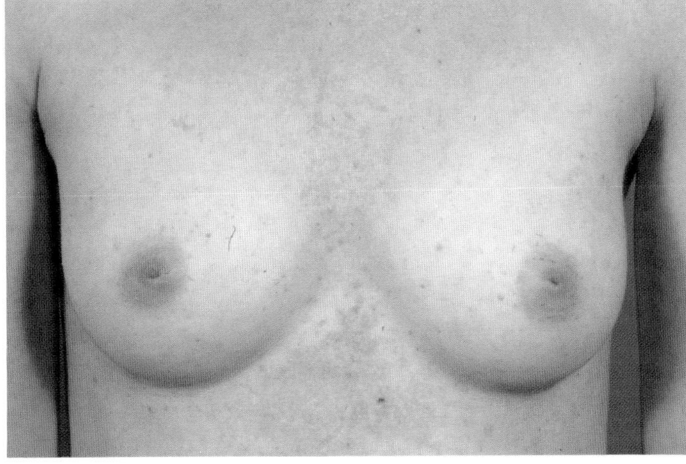

(b)

Figure 10.7

(a) Patient with Darier's disease before treatment with oral isotretinoin (1 mg/kg per day). **(b)** The same patient after treatment.

observations four patients treated with etretinate cleared completely within 14 weeks, while two untreated patients showed only slight improvement of their symptoms and still had their disease at 80 weeks.[4]

Classical adult-onset PRP is usually a self-limiting disease – 80 per cent of cases resolve within 3 years if untreated. It is a chronic skin disorder that is frequently difficult to treat and remains a disease of unknown aetiology. It has been suggested that there are decreased serum retinol-binding protein (RBP) levels in PRP patients.[5] However, Kanerva et al[1] and Stoll et al[6] both failed to show a change in serum RBP levels from normal in PRP patients.

PRP is an epidermal mildly hyperproliferative disorder, though not to the same extent as psoriasis. The epidermis usually shows slightly irregular psoriasiform hyperplasia with alternating vertical and horizontal hyper- and parakeratosis. There is an inflammatory cell infiltrate present around the

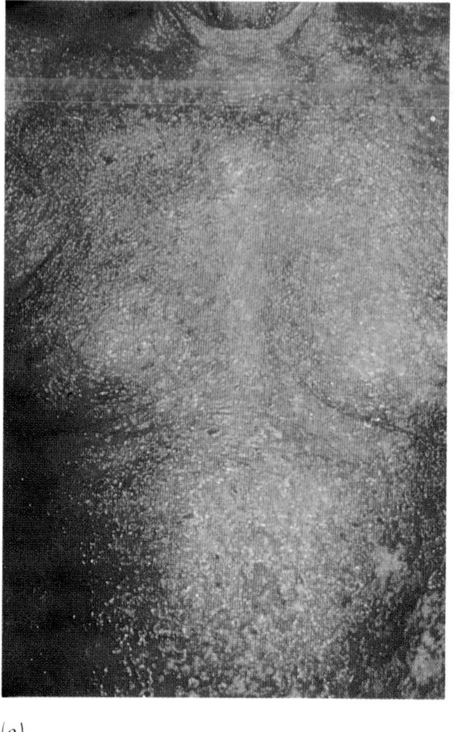
(a)

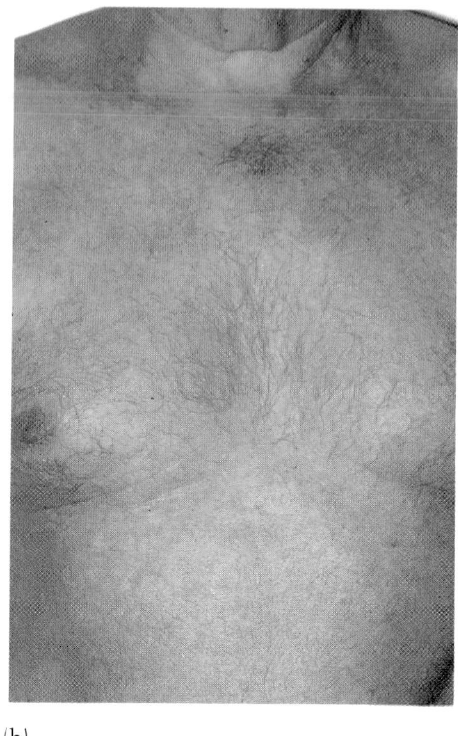
(b)

Figure 10.8

(a) Adult-onset PRP patient before treatment with etretinate 1 mg/kg per day for 6 months.
(b) The same patient after treatment.

vessels of the superficial vascular plexus, but not to the same intensity as in psoriasis. In addition, neutrophils are not prominent in the inflammatory cell infiltrate as they are in psoriasis.[7]

Other systemic treatments occasionally successful for PRP include methotrexate,[8] mega-doses of vitamin A,[9,10] isotretinoin and etretinate.[1–3,11–13] Lower doses of vitamin A have not proved to be very effective (Lowe NJ, personal observations).

The initial doses usually needed for PRP are: etretinate 1 mg/kg per day, isotretinoin 1.5 mg/kg per day and acitretin 0.75 mg/kg per day.

The mechanisms by which systemic retinoids act in PRP is unknown. It is possible there are intrinsic abnormalities of endogenous retinoid metabolism, retinoid receptor or cell transport mechanism in PRP. These abnormalities may be overcome by retinoid therapy resulting in disease remission. Etretinate appears first to decrease the hyperkeratosis and parakeratosis and then subsequently to decrease the inflammatory response. This suggests an effect on epidermal differentiation

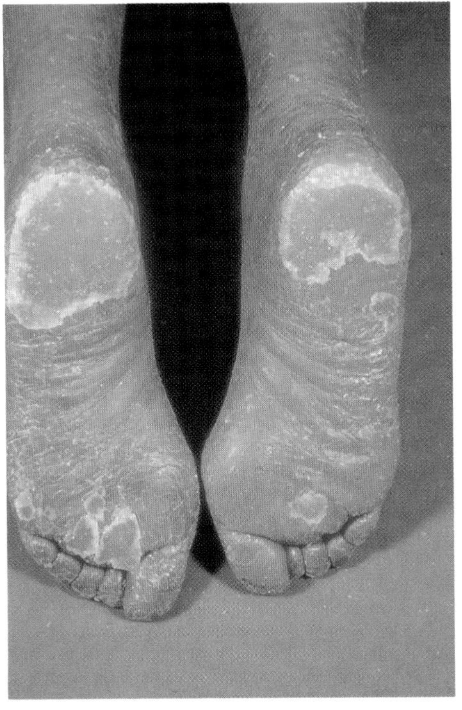

(a)

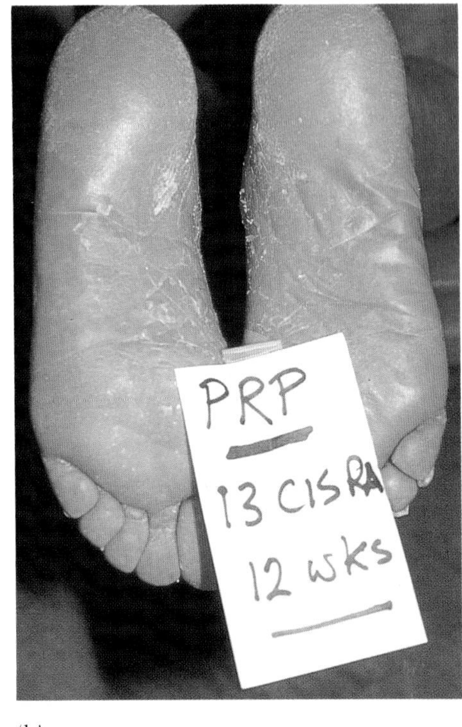

(b)

Figure 10.9

(a) Adult-onset PRP patient before treatment with isotretinoin 1.5 mg/kg per day for 3 months.
(b) The same patient after treatment.

as an early response to systemic retinoid therapy (see Figures 10.8 and 10.9).

Epidermal naevoid syndromes

A variety of epidermal naevoid syndromes may be considered for oral retinoid therapy. Examples include linear verrucous zosteriform naevi and naevus unis lateris. An example of a linear verrucous epidermal naevus patient responding to oral isotretinoin is shown in Figure 10.10.

Porokeratosis of Mibelli

This is a rare keratinocyte differentiation abnormality which may be effectively treated with etretinate or acitretin therapy. Maintenance treatment is generally required of about 25 mg p.o. daily.[14]

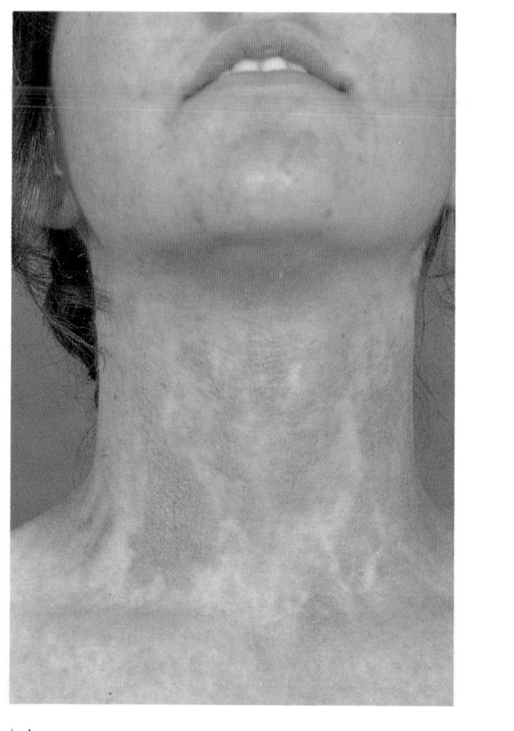

(a)

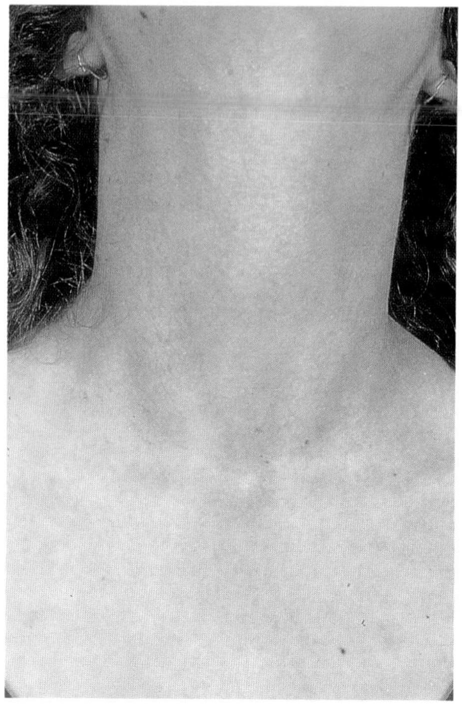

(b)

Figure 10.10

(a) Linear ichthyosiform epidermal naevus before treatment with oral isotretinoin 1 mg/kg per day. **(b)** The same patient after treatment.

Disseminated superficial actinic porokeratosis (DSAP)

In the author's experience, response of DSAP to retinoids is unpredictable.[15] Other studies report treatment failure.[16] Again maintenance with systemic or topical retinoids is often required.

Summary

Systemic retinoids have an important part to play in the treatment of various disorders of keratinization. Most of the original studies used isotretinoin[17] or etretinate. Over the last few years, experience with acitretin in the management of these disorders has expanded. The general impression is that acitretin and etretinate are comparable as regards clinical effectiveness and side-effects. They are effective at lower doses than those required for isotretinoin. In view of the pharmacological profile, the risk of teratogenicity after drug discontinuation may be somewhat less for acitretin than for etretinate, and thus acitretin may be used in women of childbearing potential providing contraceptive precautions are taken during therapy and for 1–2 years after discontinuation.

Selected skeletal radiographic studies (lateral views of spine, hips, knees and ankles) are suggested if a patient is treated for longer than 12 months or with more than 25 g of etretinate to exclude clinically significant skeletal and extraskeletal hyperostosis. The threshold doses at which skeletal changes may be expected with isotretinoin and acitretin have not been determined, but radiographic examination is suggested after 2 years of continuous therapy.

References

1. Kanerva L, Lauharanta J, Niema KM et al, Ultrastructure of pityriasis rubra pilaris with observation during retinoid treatment. *Br J Dermatol* (1981) **104**: 653–63.
2. Marks R, Finlay AY, Holt PJA, Severe disorders of keratinization: effects of treatment with Tigason (etretinate). *Br J Dermatol* (1981) **104**: 667–73.
3. Borok M, Lowe N, Further observations of systemic retinoid therapy. *J Am Acad Dermatol* (1990) **22**(5): 792–5.
4. Tabibian P, Lowe NJ, Pityriasis rubra pilaris: etretinate shortens duration of disease. *J Dermatol Treat* (1993) **4**: 9–11.
5. Finzi AF, Altomare G, Bergamaschini L et al, Pityriasis rubra pilaris and retinol-binding protein. *Br J Dermatol* (1981) **104**: 253–6.
6. Stoll DM, King LE Jr, Chytil F, Serum levels of retinol-binding protein in patients with pityriasis rubra pilaris. *Br J Dermatol* (1983) **106**: 375 (letter).
7. Soeprono F, Histologic criteria for the diagnosis of pityriasis rubra pilaris. *Am J Dermatopathol* (1986) **8**: 277–83.
8. Hanke CW, Steck WD, Childhood-onset PRP treated with methotrexate administered intravenously. *Cleve Clin Quart* (1983) **50**(2): 201–3.
9. Randle HW, Diaz-Perz JL, Winkelmann JRK, Toxic doses of vitamin A for pityriasis rubra pilaris. *Arch Dermatol* (1980) **116**: 888–92.
10. Griffiths WAD, Vitamin A and pityriasis rubra piliaris. *J Am Acad Dermatol* (1982) **7**: 555.
11. Griffiths WAD, Pitriasis rubra pilaris. *Clin Exp Dermatol* (1980) **116**: 888–92.
12. Viglioglia PA, Therapeutic evaluation of the oral retinoid RO 10-9359 in several non-psoriatic dermatoses. *Br J Dermatol* (1980) **103**: 483–7.
13. Lauharanta J, Lassus A, Treatment of pityriasis rubra pilaris with an oral aromatic retinoid (RO 10-9359). *Acta Derm Venerol (Stockh)* (1980) **60**: 460–2.
14. Bundino S, Zina AM, Disseminated Porokeratosis Mibelli treated with RO 10-9359. *Dermatologica* (1980) **160**: 328–36.
15. Ludero-Zimoch G, Rubiscz-Brezinska J, A case of disseminated superficial actinic porokeratosis. *Przegl Dermatol* (1989) **76**: 54–57.
16. Schwarz T, Seiser A, Gschnaub F, Disseminated superficial actinic porokeratosis. *J Am Acad Dermatol* (1984) **11**: 724–30.
17. Risch J, Ashton RE, Lowe NJ et al, 13-*cis*-Retinoic acid for dyskeratinizing diseases – clinicopathological responses. *Clin Exp Dermatol* (1984) **9**: 472–83.

11 Lichen planus and cutaneous lupus erythematosus

Ronald Marks

Introduction

The retinoid drugs are best known for their therapeutic effects in the major disorders of keratinization, especially the ichthyoses and Darier's disease. These agents are also now an established alternative in the treatment of stubborn psoriasis and are the major therapeutic option for the management of severe nodulocystic acne.

However, the above disorders are by no means the only ones that can be treated successfully with retinoids, and this chapter is intended to draw attention to the useful therapeutic actions of retinoids in lichen planus (LP) and cutaneous discoid lupus erythematosus (CDLE). These two disorders have several factors in common. They both appear to be the result of autoaggressive influences resulting in damage and in some cases destruction of the basal layer of the epidermis. While hypergranulosis and hyperkeratosis are predominantly features of LP, and epidermal atrophy and hyperkeratosis are notable features of CDLE, the epidermal changes in the two disorders overlap, and indeed in some cases can be quite difficult to tell apart.[1]

Although the two conditions are usually distinguished easily from the clinical point of view, LP is associated with a range of other putative autoimmune diseases[2,3] and there are a small number of patients in whom there appears to be a genuine overlap.[4] The relationship between LP and CDLE, and especially the similarities in immunopathogenesis, make it seem likely that the retinoid drugs have a similar (although as yet unknown) mode of action in these two diseases.

Lichen planus

Many papers on the benefits of topical retinoids in LP have appeared, although most have concerned the effects on oral LP. The first reports of the response of stubborn oral LP to topical tretinoin appeared in the early 1970s from Europe. Günther, Scheiber and Plewig, and Ebner reported the benefits of topical tretinoin in LP of the oral mucosa[5–9] following a series of open uncontrolled trials. A little later these highly suggestive but uncontrolled observations were supported by a controlled study by Sloberg et al.[10] This group treated 38 patients with oral mucosal LP with either 0.1% tretinoin in an adhesive base (23 patients) or with the adhesive base alone (15 patients). This trial, while not randomized or double blind, demonstrated striking benefit to the tretinoin-treated patients – 71 per cent of the patients with atrophic erosive lesions and 74 per cent of those with classical reticular lesions showed a marked response compared with 29 and 15 per cent rates for those treated with the adhesive base alone.

Giustina et al from Ann Arbor, Michigan,[11] treated 22 patients with either 0.1% isotretinoin gel or the gel vehicle alone in a randomized, double-blind, cross-over study published in 1986. The treatment with the active retinoid material lasted 2 months, and 20 of the 22 patients completed the study. The severity of the patient's lesions was classified on a 0–5 scale and those on the active retinoid application improved from a mean of 3.0 to 1.7 at 8 weeks, while the control group were virtually unchanged with mean scores of 3.6 and 3.4 at the beginning and end, respectively. Only transient local side-effects were noted and there were no systemic toxic side-effects. Unfortunately, the lesions returned after the active treatment stopped.

Topical fenretinide proved helpful in eight patients with diffuse oral lichen planus or leukoplakia. After one month's treatment two patients went into remission and six had a greater than 75 per cent response.[12]

There is little published on the response of cutaneous LP to topical tretinoin or isotretinoin (as opposed to that of mucosal LP), but our own experience suggests that this is not a particularly effective form of treatment. However, the oral retinoid drugs do seem to provide a useful therapeutic alternative in both oral and cutaneous LP. As long ago as 1975, Stüttgen[13] reported that systemic tretinoin had a therapeutic action in severe oral LP but the severe side-effects made this form of treatment impractical. Oral etretinate has been reported to be helpful in oral LP by several authors,[14,15] but the most convincing report is that of Hersle et al.[16] These workers studied 28 patients in whom the LP had been present for at least 6 months and whose clinical picture was 'compatible with LP' clinically, histologically and by immunofluorescence tests. The 28 patients were randomized to either a group receiving 75 mg etretinate daily or a group receiving identical appearing placebo. Nine patients who did not respond at the end of the 2-month trial were found to have taken the placebo and were 'crossed over' to the active medication. Those treated with etretinate showed an impressive 93 per cent improvement compared with 5 per cent improvement in the placebo-treated group. Those patients who were crossed over to receive the active substance also showed a striking improvement. Low-dose oral isotretinoin has also been reported on favourably by Strauss and Bergfeld.[17]

It is our recommendation that etretinate by mouth should be considered a first-line treatment for adults with widespread severe symptomatic cutaneous LP. In our experience most patients respond satisfactorily within 3–4 weeks and although relapse is not uncommon the condition does not appear to recur in a substantial number of subjects. Regrettably there are no hard figures in the literature to back up these anecdotal observations, and it is hoped that some will be available soon.

LP of the nails is especially difficult to treat and it was encouraging to read of a Japanese patient with LP of the nails who seemed to benefit from the use of oral etretinate alongside a steroid lotion.[18]

There are few reports of the use of oral retinoids for oral LP although their use is mentioned by Itin et al in a patient with erosive LP of the lip.[19]

We can only guess at the mode of action of retinoids in LP. We cannot even say for certain whether the topical retinoids have the same effects as the oral compounds. The modulation of epidermal repair and differentiation is certainly one possible target for the therapeutic actions of these agents in LP. Schell et al[20] studied the epidermal cell population kinetics in lichen planus using the tritiated thymidine autoradiographic labelling index technique in four patients after taking etretinate. Increased values were found after treatment but this did not seem to help the authors in reaching any reasonable explanation for the therapeutic effect. An alternative therapeutic route is via T-lymphocyte activity such as interferon release or some other aspect of the supposed immunopathogenesis of LP.

Cutaneous lupus erythematosus

Various types of CDLE are reported to have been helped by systemic retinoid drugs. The systemic forms of the disease, when present at the same time as skin lesions, do not appear to be much affected by retinoids even though the LE of the skin improves.

Uitto et al[21] and later Grupper et al[22] described groups of patients with verrucous and hypertrophic lesions of CDLE who showed excellent responses to treatment with oral etretinate in some 4–8 weeks. Ruzicka et al reported a study in which 19 CDLE patients were treated for periods of from 2 to 6 weeks with 50 mg etretinate daily.[23] When clinical response occurred the dose was reduced to 25 mg daily. Clearing occurred in eight patients and a good response in three others. Response occurred in all cases in 2–4 weeks and was apparently more notable in the male patients. It was also reported that the treatment seemed equipotent to chloroquine and could be combined with either topical or systemic corticosteroids.

Ruzicka et al later described the treatment of 20 CDLE patients with acitretin[24] in whom the diagnosis had been confirmed by histology and immunofluorescence. The patients were treated for a maximum of 12 weeks, but the acitretin was stopped if there was no response at 6 weeks. Acitretin was given at an initial dose of 50 mg and adjusted to the response (10–75 mg). Interestingly, all patients seemed to improve, but in five the response was less than satisfactory, requiring a change of therapy. Seven patients showed 'complete' clearing and five of these had subacute CDLE (out of six who had this type of LE in the entire group). The authors were particularly impressed with the excellent response of two female patients with severe recalcitrant CDLE. There did not appear to be any serious side-effects or any worsening of the laboratory findings of LE.

The same group reported the results of a multicentre, randomized, double-blind, clinical trial in which acitretin (50 mg/day) was compared with hydroxychloroquine (400 mg/day) in 28 and 30 patients respectively over an 8-week period. Overall improvement occurred in 13 of 28 treated with acitretin compared with 15 of 30 patients treated with hydroxychloroquine. Although there were more side-effects with acitretin it is clear that both treatments are useful in different patients.[25]

Isotretinoin was used to treat ten patients with CDLE in a study by Newton et al.[26] Eight of these ten patients completed a 16-week course of 80 mg isotretinoin daily and showed an excellent response clinically. The stated intention of the study was to identify the mechanism of action of isotretinoin in this disorder and all manner of investigations were performed before and after treatment, including histopathology, direct immunofluorescence, electron microscopy, and tissue immunophenotyping of lymphyocytes as well as determination of lymphocyte subsets in the peripheral blood. No dramatic alterations were detected which could give a clue to the primary mode of action of isotretinoin, although the expected improvement in histology occurred *pari passu* with the clinical improvement. Other reports of the efficacy of isotretinoin include two in which individual patients with severe recalcitrant hypertrophic and warty lesions were treated. Both patients had lesions that were at one stage interpreted as being keratoacanthomas. One patient

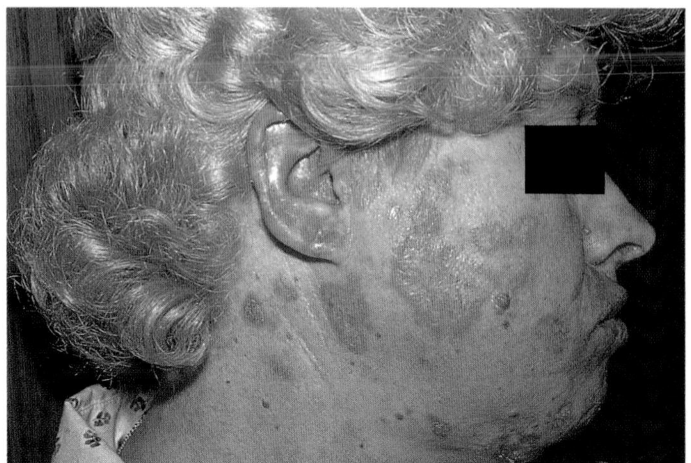

Figure 11.1

A 40-year-old woman with long-standing chronic discoid lupus erythematosus **(a)** before and **(b)** after 6 months of 25 mg etretinate daily. (Courtesy of NJ Lowe, MD.)

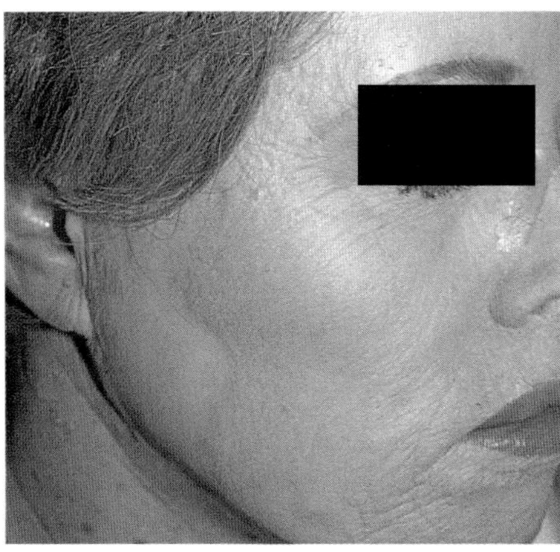

(b)

responded to the isotretinoin alone and the other responded to a combination of hydroxy-chloroquine and isotretinoin.

Our own experience is with etretinate predominantly (Figure 11.1). There can be little doubt that the majority of patients show a gratifying response with tolerable side-effects. Sadly the lesions recur after treatment is stopped in most patients, but often can be controlled with a relatively small dose of retinoid and can be maintained till remission occurs – as it usually does. As yet special investigations have not identified the mode of action of the retinoid drugs in CDLE. The patient shown in Figure 11.1 has been well controlled for 3 years on low-dosage etretinate; her current dosage is 25 mg orally on alternate days, plus daily sunscreens.

Conclusion

Both LP and CDLE are improved by treatment with oral retinoid drugs. In LP improvement also occurs with topical retinoids, although most of the documented successes are with the oral form of the disease. As yet there is no information as to whether these drugs act on the epidermal, the inflammatory components or both elements of these disorders.

References

1. Davies MG, Gorkiewicz A, Knight A et al, Is there a relationship between lupus erythematosus and lichen planus? *Br J Dermatol* (1977) **96**: 145–54.
2. Shuttleworth D, Graham-Brown RAC, Campbell AC, The autoimmune background in lichen planus. *Br J Dermatol* (1986) **115**: 199–203.
3. Cerimele D, Lichen planus and internal medicine. *Ital Gen Rev Dermatol* (1988) **25**: 41–166.
4. Van der Horst JC, Cirkel PKS, Neiboer C, Mixed lichen planus–lupus erythematosus disease – a distinct entity? Clinical histopathological and immunopathological studies in six patients. *Clin Exp Dermatol* (1983) **8**: 631–40.
5. Günther S, Vitamin A acid treatment of oral lichen planus. *Arch Dermatol* (1973) **107**: 277.
6. Günther S, The therapeutic value of retinoic acid (vitamin A acid) in lichen planus of the oral mucous membrane. *Dermatologica* (1973) **147**: 130–6.
7. Günther S, ber Wirksamkeit der Vitamin-A-Säure bei Erkrankungen der Mundschleimhaut: Lichen ruber planus, Leukoplakien und Lingua geographica. *Z Hautkr* (1975) **50**: 41.
8. Scheiber W, Plewig G, Behandlung des Lichen ruber mucosae mit Vitamin-A-Säure-Derivaten. *Dermatologica* (1978) **157**: 171–80.
9. Ebner H, Miescher P, Raff M, Lokalbehundlung des Lichen ruber planus der Mundschleimhaut mit Vitamin-A-Säure. *Z Hautkr* (1974) **48**: 735–40.
10. Sloberg K, Hersel K, Mobacken H et al, Topical vitamin A acid and oral lichen planus. *Arch Dermatol* (1979) **115**: 716–18.
11. Giustina TS, Stewart JCB, Ellis CN et al, Topical application of isotretinoin gel improves oral lichen planus. *Arch Dermatol* (1986) **122**: 534–6.
12. Trodati N, Chiesa F, Rossi N et al, *Cancer Lett* (1994) **76**: 109–11.
13. Stüttgen G, Oral vitamin A acid therapy. *Acta Derm Venereol (Stcokh)* (1975) **55** (suppl 74): 174–9.
14. Maidhof R, Zur systemischen Behandlung des oralen Lichen planus mit einem aromatischen Retinoid (Ro 10-9359). *Z Hautkr* (1979) **54**: 873–6.
15. Schuppli R, The efficacy of a new retinoid (Ro 10-9359). *Z Hautkr* (1970) **54**: 873–6.
16. Hersle K, Mobacken H, Sloberg K et al, Severe oral lichen planus: treatment with an aromatic retinoid (etretinate). *Br J Dermatol* (1982) **106**: 77–80.
17. Strauss ME, Bergfeld WF, Treatment of oral lichen planus with low-dose isotretinoin. *J Am Acad Dermatol* (1984) **11**: 527–8.
18. Kato N, Ueno H, Isolated lichen planus of the nails treated with etretinate. *J Dermatol* (1993) **20**: 577–80.
19. Itin PH, Schiller P, Gilli L, Buechner SA, Isolated LP of the Lip. *Br J Dermatol* (1995) **132**: 1000–2.
20. Schell A, Hornstein PQP, Deinlein E et al, Epithelial cell proliferation of oral lichen planus in patients treated with an aromatic retinoid. *Acta Derm Venereol (Stockh)* (1983) **63**: 66–8.
21. Uitto J, Santa Cruz DJ, Eisen AZ et al, Verrucous lesions in patients with discoid lupus erythematosus. *Br J Dermatol* (1978) **98**: 507–20.
22. Grupper CH, Berretti B, Lupus erythematosus and etretinate. In: WJ Cunliffe, AJ Miller (eds). *Retinoid therapy*. Springer-Verlag: New York, 1984, pp 73–81.
23. Ruzicka R, Meurer M, Braun-Falco O, Treatment of cutaneous lupus erythematosus with etretinate. *Acta Derm Venereol (Stockh)* (1985) **65**: 324–9.
24. Ruzicka R, Meurer M, Bieber T, Efficiency of acitretin in the treatment of cutaneous lupus erythematosus. *Arch Dermatol* (1988) **124**: 897–902.
25. Ruzicka T, Sommerburg C, Goerz G et al, Treatment of cutaneous lupus erythematous with acitretin and hydroxychloroquine. *Br J Dermatol* (1992) **127**: 513–8.
26. Newton RC, Jorizzo JL, Solomon AR et al, Mechanism-oriented assessment of isotretinoin in chronic or subacute cutaneous lupus erythematosus. *Arch Dermatol* (1986) **122**: 170–6.

12 Toxicity

Nicholas J Lowe and Michael David

Introduction

The toxic side-effects from the therapeutic use of retinoids closely resemble the hypervitaminosis A syndrome.[1] Their incidence and severity are usually dose related and reversible upon withdrawal of the drug. Hypersensitivity reactions are extremely rare. Acute retinoid toxicities are observed mainly on the skin and mucous membranes. Serious toxic side-effects include teratogenicity, effects on the metabolism of lipids and changes in liver function. However, accumulating clinical data indicate that their chronic toxicity particularly involves the skeletal system.

The toxicity spectrum of retinoids varies with the analogue being tested.[2] For example, etretinate seems to be less toxic than isotretinoin in respect of photosensitivity, alterations in lipid metabolism and influence on the central nervous system, whereas acitretin may be less toxic to bones than etretinate. Arotinoid ethyl may not influence serum lipid levels. These differences should be recognized by the clinician, because they can influence the selection of a retinoid for treatment.

Systemic retinoids

Systemic administration of retinoids is frequently associated with mucocutaneous side-effects, liver toxicity and abnormalities of the serum lipid profile. Currently, the main factors limiting more common use of retinoids are their teratogenicity and chronic bone toxicity. Treatment with retinoids requires appropriate selection of patients, careful periodic monitoring of the clinical response, and appropriate laboratory tests. Careful therapeutic management is necessary in order to prevent or minimize side-effects.

Mucocutaneous toxicity

Almost all patients receiving a retinoid complain of dryness of the lips; less than 30 per cent manifest dryness of the mouth. Clinical observation reveals chapped lips with excessive desquamation and fissures. Xerosis of the nasal mucosa is associated with nasal bleeding in less than 15 per cent of patients and is probably due to thinning and hyperfragility of the mucosa.[3–6]

Colonization of the nares with *Staphylococcus aureus* with subsequent infection has been reported in patients taking isotretinoin[7] or etretinate.[8] Antibiotic prophylaxis is recommended in patients with cardiac valve disease during oral retinoid treatment. No specific toxic side-effects have been recorded on the anogenital mucosae.

The most common cutaneous side-effects include xerosis of the skin, frequently associated with pruritus and sometimes with erythema and skin hyperfragility and desquamation, particularly of the palms and soles.[4,6,9] Retinoid dermatitis, that is, the appearance of an erythematous, papular rash mimicking psoriasis, mycosis fungoides,[10] pityriasis rosacea or eczema craquelé,[11] has been reported (Figure 12.1). The last of these conditions, especially, may reflect the drying effect of the drug. Generalization of these symptoms over the entire body can lead to erythroderma, although this is very rare.[12] The slight erythema and stratum corneum alterations may partly explain the shiny, smooth appearance of the skin. The so-called sticky skin associated with retinoid treatment may be due to increased glycoprotein deposition.

Patients on etretinate may feel cold even on warm days and sometimes develop chills as a result of excessive loss of heat through the erythematous skin.

Photosensitivity is an occasional adverse reaction to the use of retinoids. An increased susceptibility to sunburn has been reported in association with isotretinoin and etretinate therapy in 7–12 per cent of patients. However, phototesting of subjects receiving etretinate or isotretinoin fails to produce evidence of an abnormal minimum erythema dose.[13,14] Photosensitivity attributable to etretinate is rare.[15] Combined use of etretinate and PUVA or ultraviolet B is popular for psoriatic patients. Moreover, we encourage patients receiving etretinate to expose their skin to sunlight and have never seen photosensitivity reaction. In vitro photohaemolysis studies by Ferguson and Johnson have shown that tretinoin, isotretinoin and acitretin are potentially phototoxic, whereas etretinate is not. Whether photosensitivity results from an idiosyncratic reaction, perhaps secondary to altered pharmocokinetics, or to increased desquamation causing thinning of the stratum corneum and loss of the photoprotective property of the horny layer, remains uncertain. Facial erythema (Figure 12.2) occurs in some 50 per cent of acne patients receiving isotretinoin and is sometimes associated with a transient flare of the acne.[3,16] To what extent this facial dermatitis might be related to photosensitivity is unclear.

Palmoplantar papulopustular lesions have been observed in patients after institution of etretinate therapy.[17] In one report, it was suggested that these lesions result from a retinoid-induced palmoplantar miliaria in hyperhidrotic patients.[18] It has also been speculated that the small papules represent an early stage of the psoriasis lesions.

Some rare skin manifestations have been reported in association with retinoid treatment. A nodular prurigo-like eruption[19] occurred in two patients receiving etretinate. A rosacea-like eruption and generalized oedema associated with etretinate[20] have also been observed. However, in the latter cases, the aetiological relationship to etretinate is doubtful since the patients had renal failure.

Allergic drug eruptions from retinoids are extremely rare. We had the opportunity to observe erythema multiforme that appeared shortly after commencement of etretinate treatment in two patients. The aetiological relationship was confirmed in one patient by rechallenge (unpublished data). It seems that under normal circumstances retinoid molecules lack antigenic properties.

There have been several case reports of vasculitis as a side-effect of oral retinoids, particularly isotretinoin. The temporal relationships and the number of reports suggest that vasculitis is a rare but true toxic side-effect from the use of oral retinoids. A case of

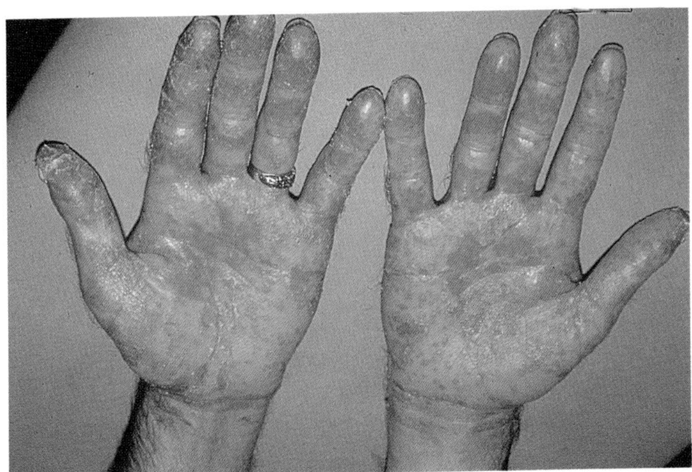

Figure 12.1

Severe retinoid dermatitis of hands in patient on etretinate for psoriasis.

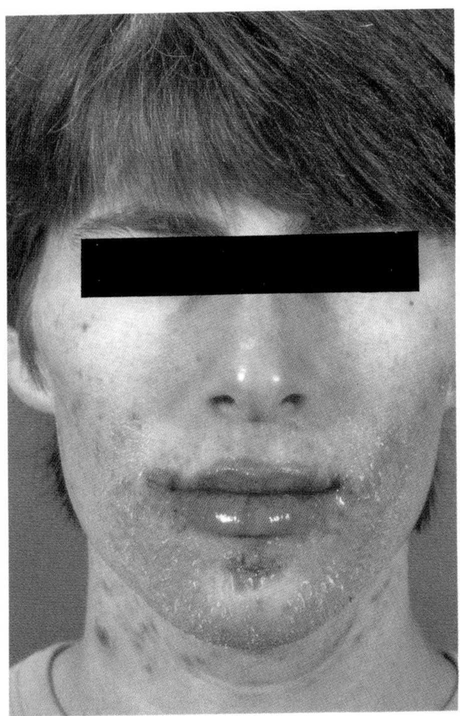

Figure 12.2

Patient with facial dermatitis induced in isotretinoin 1 mg/kg per day.

Wegener's granulomatosis has also been recorded.

Acute retinoid toxicity may involve skin adnexae, namely hair and nails. Etretinate, acitretin and, to a lesser extent, isotretinoin cause diffuse hair loss in 10–25 per cent of patients.[21,22,23] It is uncommon for this to be severe, but in women this reaction is one of the reasons for discontinuation of therapy. It appears to be due to shortening of the anagen phase of the cell cycle. The hair loss is related directly to the dosage and is reversible when the drug is withdrawn. Patients may complain that the hair becomes thin. Interestingly, the shape and physical properties of the new hair are different from those of the hair before retinoid treatment. For example, it sometimes becomes permanently curly, kinked[24] or twisted.[25] The most common site of hair loss is the scalp, but some patients manifest loss of eyebrow or eyelash hair.

Many patients develop nail changes during retinoid treatment. The common changes include loss of the glistening and shiny appearance of the nails, which may become thin, fragile, and soft, and may eventually loosen and fall off.[26] The dystrophic changes

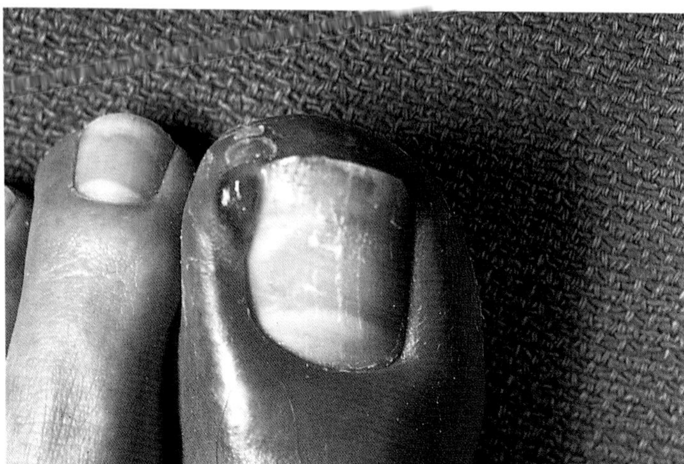

Figure 12.3

Severe paronychial pyogenic granuloma in patient on etretinate.

of the nail may coexist with redness and swelling of the skin fold around the nail, so-called paronychia-like changes.[27] Excessive granulation tissue round the nails may occur without associated nail dystrophy.[27,28] The formation of excessive granulation tissue and the occurrence of pyogenic granuloma-like lesions in patients with nodular acne (Figure 12.3) probably represent the same phenomenon.[29] Two cases of pyogenic granuloma-like lesions have also been reported during etretinate treatment.[30] A direct effect of the drugs on fibroblasts and endothelial cells may explain these observations.[27,31]

We and others have observed patients with increased formation of cerumen in the external ear, otitis externa[32] and earache.[33]

Some of the common mucocutaneous side-effects may be relieved by topical applications of emollients and lubricating agents. For more severe cheilitis or dermatitis, hydrocortisone ointment is often beneficial. The use of topical antibiotics for the nose and eyes is helpful for reduction of bacterial proliferation. Paronychia-like reactions and excessive periungual granulation tissue are resistant to topical treatment; however, steroid therapy by occlusive dressing or intralesional injection may be helpful.

Ocular toxicity

Eye toxicities involve the conjunctival membrane, cornea and retina. Isotretinoin has been detected in tears following treatment,[34] so the ocular surface is exposed to the drug via the tear film. Subjective symptoms include dryness, irritation, pain and, on rare occasions, night blindness.[35] The dryness of the conjunctiva caused by diminished tear secretion may interfere with the patient's ability to wear contact lenses.[36] Blepharitis and conjunctivitis occur in 20–45 per cent of treated patients.[37] *Staphylococcus aureus* has been cultured from the eyelids of individuals taking isotretinoin.[38] Blepharoconjunctivitis is more commonly due to isotretinoin than to etretinate.[22] If cases develop, manifested by discomfort or pain in the eye, frequent application of artificial tears or a lubricating preparation is very useful. Eleven patients with corneal opacities and three patients with optic atrophy possibly related to retinoid treatment were found among 237 individuals with eye complaints.[36]

There have recently been reports of defective vision in patients treated with isotretinoin and the experimental retinoid fenretinide.[35,39] Isotretinoin induced abnormal night vision in 3 of 50 patients. The clinical symptoms were confirmed by abnormal dark-adaption curves, electroretinograms (ERGs) and electro-oculograms.[39] In a prospective study, two of six patients showed deterioration in scotopic ERG during treatment with isotretinoin.[40] Recently, two of eight psoriatic patients treated with fenretinide developed symptomatic night blindness, which improved approximately 3 months after stopping the drug.[35,41] Reversible abnormal rod photoreceptor function has been described in two of five patients receiving fenretinide for multiple basal cell carcinoma. This phenomenon differs from isotretinoin-induced blindness, in which recovery after discontinuation of treatment is slow and incomplete. Transient acute myopia developed on three separate occasions in a woman receiving isotretinoin.[42] Whereas acute myopia is probably an idiosyncratic reaction, night blindness may result from inhibition of one of the steps in the visual cycle normally mediated by endogenous retinoids. There is, in addition, a single case report of an individual treated with etretinate who developed abnormal function of both rods and cones which severely compromised visual acuity. Luckily vision improved after stopping the etretinate.[43]

Musculoskeletal toxicity

Some 16 per cent of patients treated with isotretinoin develop myalgia and muscle stiffness[44] and there have been rare cases of increased creatine kinase activity.[45] It has been claimed that potentiation of increased serum creatine kinase values may occur in exercising patients receiving isotretinoin.[46] Reversible skeletal muscle damage induced by isotretinoin has been described in two acne patients. The muscle symptoms appeared shortly after initiation of treatment; the histological and ultrastructural findings in one of the patients were unique and indicative of muscular and myoneural functional damage.[47]

True muscle damage induced by etretinate appears to be rare. One report mentioned elevation of creatine kinase in two patients,[48] and a single case report described increased muscle tone during etretinate therapy.[49] Recently, muscle symptoms appearing after several months of therapy were described in three psoriatic patients. There was histological and ultrastructural evidence of damage in a pattern suggestive of segmental muscle necrosis.[50]

Etretinate may cause subclinical muscle damage after long-term use as shown electromyographically by low-amplitude action potentials. Neuromuscular evaluation should be performed before and after treatment with retinoids to study this reaction further. Management of musculoskeletal side-effects includes avoidance of physical activity and administration of analgesics, myorelaxants, or both in severely affected patients.

An understanding of the signs and symptoms of hypervitaminosis A syndrome is very helpful in predicting long-term toxicity due to synthetic retinoids. Bony changes are a recognized common adverse reaction seen in chronic vitamin A intoxication. These changes include hyperostosis,[51] periostosis, demineralization, thinning of the bones and premature closure of the epiphyses.[52]

Short-term retinoid therapy in children seems to be safe as far as bone toxicity is concerned, but data concerning long-term therapy are sometimes conflicting and even contradictory. Early reports describing etretinate therapy in children[53] for 11–17 months[30] and 16–42 months[54,55] and isotretinoin treatment for 20 months[56] are encouraging. The data suggest that retinoid therapy does not interfere with development and growth, although regular monitoring of growth rate is necessary. Furthermore, Brun and Baran reported no growth or bone abnormalities after 7 years of etretinate therapy.[57] Recently, Glover et al examined 19 children and adolescents on long-term (median 5 years) etretinate treatment and found no significant bone abnormalities.[58] Mills and Marks also report experience of etretinate treatment in 12 children treated for periods of up to 10 years.[59] None of these had developed significant bone abnormalities.

In contrast to these data, several reports suggest chronic bone toxicity in children. Milstone et al described partial closure of epiphyses, demineralization, and altered bone remodelling in a 10½-year-old boy treated with 3.5 mg/kg per day isotretinoin for nearly 5 years. This boy had also received vitamin A and D supplementation after the first year of treatment.[60] Premature ephiphyseal closure was reported in two children receiving etretinate therapy for 5 and 6 years. One of them also had thinning of the long bones and two fractures after minor trauma. Osteoporosis secondary to isotretinoin treatment despite normal serum levels of calcium phosphate, vitamin D metabolites and parathormone was reported by McGuire et al.[61]

Evaluation of clinical reports of children treated with retinoids suggests that the occurrence of bone abnormalities, particularly premature closure of the epiphyses, is associated with treatment for more than 5 years, high retinoid doses and vitamin A supplementation. In our opinion, chronic treatment of children with retinoids should be undertaken only after consideration of the benefit–risk ratio by the clinician and the parents. It must be emphasized that should bone abnormalities occur, they may not resolve upon cessation of the drug.

Chronic retinoid toxicity confined to bones has been reported in adult patients treated with isotretinoin and etretinate. Pittsley and Yuoder in 1983[62] and Gerber et al in 1984[63] reported skeletal hyperostoses and anterior spinal ligament calcification in patients treated with high-dose isotretinoin for 2 years or longer. The bony abnormalities were similar to those seen in diffuse idiopathic skeletal hyperostosis (DISH). Changes occurred in the cervical spine more often than in the thoracic and lumbar spine (Figure 12.4). Isotretinoin therapy for 9 months to 1 year at a dose of 2 mg/kg has been associated with small asymptomatic hyperostoses of the spine.[64,65] In a recent prospective study, small spurs at the anterior margin of the vertebrae were seen in

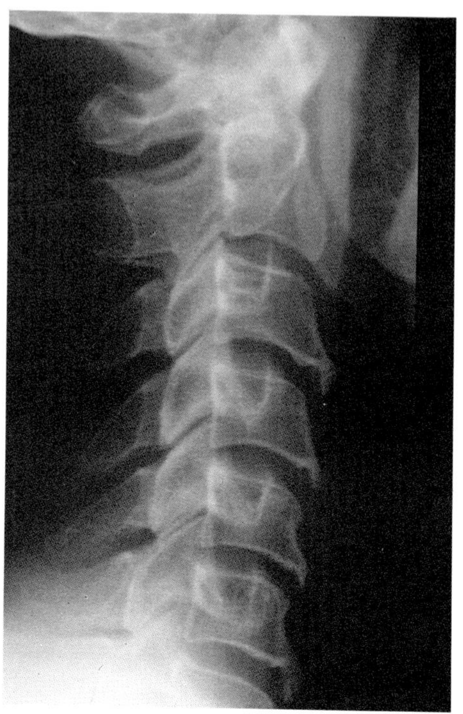

Figure 12.4

Spinal hyperostosis: Darier's disease patient treated with isotretinoin for 3 years, followed by etretinate for 5 years.

10 of 96 patients receiving short-term low-dose isotretinoin therapy.[66] In addition to spinal involvement, some patients have shown extraspinal calcification.[67] DiGiovanna et al were able to demonstrate extraspinal tendon and ligament calcification in 11 of 12 patients receiving isotretinoin for 21–105 months. The ankles, pelvis and knees were primarily involved.[68]

Early reports concerning the potential toxic effects of etretinate therapy on the skeleton failed to prove an association.[65] Gilbert et al reported an absence of skeletal radiographic changes during 6–18 months of etretinate therapy in eight psoriatic patients.[69] Although several reports described a few patients with etretinate-related bone changes,[70,71] the frequency of this adverse reaction was initially underestimated. It was DiGiovanna et al in 1986 who confirmed the association of long-term etretinate therapy with skeletal abnormalities. Of 38 patients who had received etretinate therapy for 5 years, 84 per cent had radiographic findings of extraspinal tendon and ligament calcification with frequent involvement of the ankles, pelvis and bones, and 29 per cent had spine involvement resembling DISH.[72] A prospective study of 15 patients treated with etretinate for up to 5 years did not demonstrate any bony changes by either radiological or radionuclide scanning techniques.[59] Skeletal hyperostosis is more likely to occur at etretinate cumulative doses over 30 g.[73]

There may be some doubt about the results of those of the above studies retrospectively including psoriatic patients whose spine radiographs were likely to have been abnormal before therapy, or of those involving older patients in whom bone degeneration may already have been present. However, it seems reasonable to conclude that long-term (more than 2 years) therapy with isotretinoin or etretinate will result in hyperostotic changes, and ligament and tendon calcification, or both, in most patients.

Of interest is the observation that radiographic findings correlate poorly with the presence of bone and joint symptoms, mainly pain and stiffness. About 50 per cent of patients are asymptomatic in areas of radiographic changes and, conversely, some patients have symptoms in areas that are radiographically normal. They also correlate poorly with functional changes although there are a few case reports of serious disability due to ligamentous ossification. One patient had symptoms and signs of spinal cord compression owing to changes in the vertebral column[74] and another had difficulty with the pronation–supination movement owing to calcification in the interosseous membrane in the forearm.[75]

Although the severity of bone abnormalities is related to dose and duration of treatment, the incidence of these changes correlates poorly with these factors. Minor skeletal hyperostosis can occur after moderate-dose[67] and short-term isotretinoin therapy.[64]

Unlike other retinoid toxicities, which are usually reversible upon withdrawal of the drug, it seems unlikely that hyperostosis and calcification will resolve after stopping treatment. However, no studies have addressed this issue. It is also uncertain whether low-dose (<0.5 mg/kg) or intermittent treatment is associated with less chronic toxicity or perhaps can reverse minor toxic symptoms.

Because the ankle is the most common site of involvement (Figure 12.5), it is reasonable to obtain a single radiograph of the ankle before treatment and then yearly. If ankle findings are abnormal or if other local radiographs show changes, a full radiographic view of the lateral aspect of the spine, the pelvis and the knees should be done for comprehensive assessment of bone changes.

A recent report of 20 patients treated with systemic isotretinoin for acne over 20 weeks did not report any evidence of bone demineralization.[76] Other studies have suggested that oral retinoids used chronically may have an effect on bone demineralization.[77]

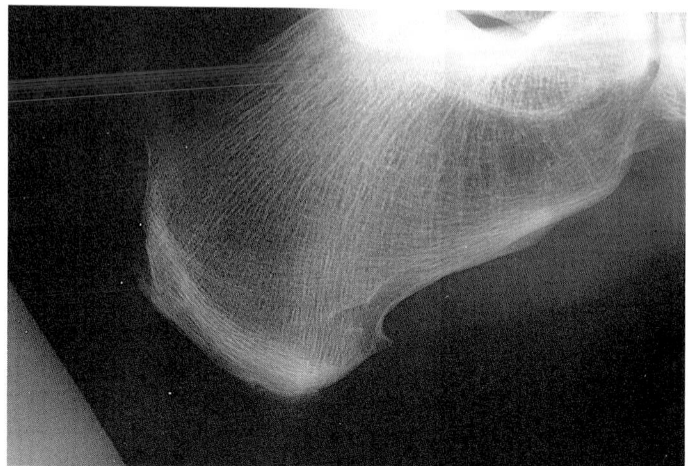
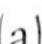

(a)

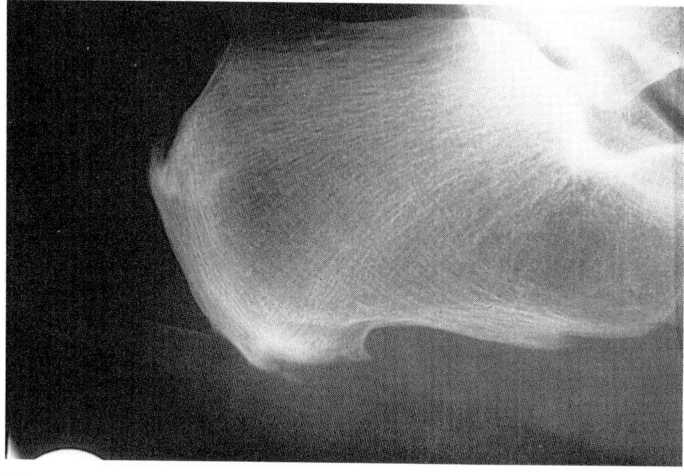

(b)

Figure 12.5

Progression of calcaneal spurs in patient on etretinate therapy for severe psoriasis. **(a)** Early in treatment; **(b)** after treatment with etretinate for 7 years – approximately 40 g cumulative etretinate.

Neurological toxicity

Pseudotumor cerebri (benign intracranial hypertension), a condition in which there is an increase in intracranial pressure and papilloedema, has been reported as occurring during isotretinoin and etretinate therapy.[36,78] In a survey of 237 patients who manifested eye symptoms while receiving isotretinoin, 18 were observed to have papilloedema; in seven of these pseudotumor cerebri syndrome eventually developed.[36] Persistent headache with abnormal vision should raise the suspicion of this syndrome, which requires immediate ophthalmological examination. In some cases of pseudotumor cerebri, isotretinoin had been given together with tetracycline or minocycline, which are also known to cause this complication. Therefore it is recommended that combined therapy with retinoids and tetracyclines be avoided. Interestingly, an attempt to commit suicide by ingestion of 800 mg isotretinoin resulted in headache, hallucinations and vertebral pain that lasted for 32 hours.[79]

Other infrequent symptoms are depression, loss of equilibrium and general malaise.[80] The question of depression,[81] a not infrequent complication of treatment with isotretinoin, has recently been discussed extensively and is at present still undecided.

Liver toxicity

Synthetic retinoids have much less affinity for the liver than does vitamin A. However, etretinate concentrates in the liver in a high tissue-to-blood ratio,[82] and indeed, most reported retinoid-induced hepatotoxic reactions, have occurred with etretinate treatment.

Liver damage caused by retinoids is a result of an acute toxic reaction.[83] The incidence of chronic liver toxicity is still uncertain. Acute changes in liver enzymes occur in 20–30 per cent of patients, usually within 0.5–2 months after commencing therapy. Transient increases of aspartate transaminase, alanine transaminase and, occasionally, lactic dehydrogenase, gamma-glutamyl transpeptidase and alkaline phosphatase have been recorded. Elevation of transaminases is mild to moderate and usually resolves in spite of continued therapy or after reduction of the dosage.[84,85] Marked alterations in liver enzymes are rare, occurring in only about 1 per cent of patients.[4] Severe acute hepatotoxic reactions probably represent idiosyncratic responses.[86,87] In one patient acute hepatitis was associated with fever and eosinophilia, suggesting a hypersensitivity reaction.[88] A case of biopsy-proven hepatitis during oral etretinate treatment has recently been reported. Hepatotoxicity did not reappear when isotretinoin was substituted for the etretinate.[89] Additional cases of acute hepatitis in association with etretinate therapy have been supported by liver biopsy findings. All patients were women, and the interval between the start of etretinate therapy and appearance of hepatitis ranged from 2 weeks to 6 months.[21,59,87]

To quantify the probability of chronic toxicity, liver biopsy studies have been performed by Zachariae et al[90] and van Voorst et al[91] who investigated a total of 54 patients on long-term (up to 6 years) therapy with retinoids. No evidence of toxicity could be confirmed. Roenigk prospectively studied 17 psoriatic patients with an increased risk of hepatotoxicity. Extensive evaluation of liver function and histological changes, including electron microscopic examination, did not reveal significant liver damage after 3 years of etretinate treatment.[92] Recently, Camuto et al studied liver morphology and function in 18 patients receiving etretinate for 5 years.[93] Mildly elevated liver enzymes were noted occasionally. Liver biopsy specimens showed moderate periportal fibrosis in two patients; one had changes similar to those of chronic active hepatitis and one had severe cirrhosis unrelated to alcohol ingestion. The authors suggested that periodic liver biopsies be performed to monitor patients on long-term etretinate. Considering that mild structural liver abnormalities may be found in psoriatic patients, many of whom have a history of intake of methotrexate or non-steroidal anti-inflammatory agents or of alcoholism, it will be difficult to prove retinoid-related chronic hepatotoxicity. Assessment of the hepatotoxic effect of etretinate requires comparison of pre-treatment and post-treatment biopsy specimens. However, in our opinion, current data are not in favour of routine liver biopsy.

Two recent reports concerning the short-term efficacy and toxicity of acitretin showed that treatment of psoriatic patients for 6 months was associated with mild aberrations of liver enzymes.[94,95] Long-term therapy with acitretin (up to 2 years) was not associated with increased liver toxicity. However, no liver biopsies have been done on patients receiving long-term therapy.

Lipid abnormalities

Hyperlipidaemia is one of the most common of the acute toxicities of synthetic retinoids. The increase in serum triglycerides and cholesterol is proportional to the dose of the drug and reverses within 4–8 weeks after stopping the retinoid.[96,97] Although retinoid-induced hyperlipidaemia is most likely to occur in patients with predisposing factors such as obesity, alcoholism, diabetes and familial hyperlipidaemia,[98] the increase in serum lipids is not related to the pre-treatment levels.[97,99] The incidence of retinoid-induced hyperlipidaemia varies among studies.

Isotretinoin-induced hypertriglyceridaemia probably occurs in approximately 35 per cent of patients, higher than most estimates; hypercholesterolaemia probably occurs in 30–40 per cent. A similar frequency of lipid abnormalities has been reported with etretinate.[97,100]

Ultracentrifugation studies have demonstrated that, during isotretinoin therapy, the greatest increase in triglycerides is associated with the very-low-density lipoprotein (VLDL) fraction, with a smaller increase in low-density lipoprotein (LDL) triglycerides and high-density lipoprotein (HDL) triglycerides.[97,101] The HDL triglycerides do not change with etretinate therapy. During isotretinoin therapy, the greatest increase in cholesterol is associated with LDL, with a smaller increase in VLDL cholesterol and a decrease in HDL cholesterol.

Conflicting findings have been published with regard to alterations of cholesterol during etretinate therapy. For example, some studies suggest that the increase in VLDL cholesterol is greater than the increase in LDL cholesterol,[98] while other studies have reported the increase to be limited to the LDL fraction.[97] HDL cholesterol has been found by some investigators to be decreased slightly by etretinate, but no differences have been found by others.[100] Both isotretinoin and etretinate induce increases in VLDL and LDL detected by lipoprotein electrophoresis. Increased concentrations of apoprotein B,[97,98] a small increase in total apoprotein A[98] and no changes in the levels of apoprotein A1 and apoprotein A2 have been reported after etretinate and isotretinoin therapy.[97]

Short-term therapy with acitretin induces a slight elevation of triglycerides and cholesterol in about 35 and 30 per cent of patients, respectively. However, only a few patients require dose adjustment. We have followed a group of 15 patients receiving acitretin for 2 years. After an initial increase in triglyceride and cholesterol levels, there was a decrease or at least a stabilization in serum lipid values. This second change might be attributed to dietary modification and administration of fish oil capsules.

In a preliminary study, arotinoid ethyl ester has been shown to possess a clinical efficacy and toxicity profile similar to that of etretinate but without an effect on serum lipid levels.[102] Additional study is needed to confirm this potential advantage.

Among the several possible explanations for retinoid-induced hyperlipidaemia, enhanced synthesis of lipoproteins may be the most likely.[103] The higher levels of apoproteins after treatment with retinoids support this concept. Increased lipid synthesis is another possibility.[103] A recent study showed no change in the level of serum non-esterified fatty acids in patients treated with isotretinoin,[104] which led the authors to suggest that hyperlipidaemia induced by isotretinoin may be attributable to an increase in circulating lipoproteins caused by increased production or impaired catabolism.

Severe hypertrigylceridaemia may be associated with eruptive xanthomas and acute haemorrhagic pancreatitis. Indeed, hypertriglyceridaemia with a value above 4000 mg/dl and eruptive xanthomas were reported in one patient given 2.5 mg/kg per day isotretinoin for Darier's disease.[105] Acute haemorrhagic pancreatitis associated with isotretinoin therapy has also been described.[16]

Whereas short-term therapy with retinoids seems unlikely to increase the risk of coronary heart disease, this possibility may exist with chronic retinoid therapy.[106] Because of the increased LDL cholesterol and decreased HDL cholesterol in patients receiving long-term retinoid therapy, the possibility of accelerated arteriosclerosis and an increased risk of coronary heart disease are a matter of concern. Periodic measurements of lipid levels in patients receiving retinoids are mandatory. Furthermore, the percentage of HDL cholesterol and the LDL/HDL ratio may be useful for predicting an increased risk of cardiac disease.[106]

Increased levels of triglycerides and cholesterol during retinoid treatment can be managed at least partially by an appropriate diet and supplementation with fish oil capsules (omega-3 fatty acids). In a double-blind study, Marsden demonstrated a significant reduction in the triglyceride and cholesterol levels increased by isotretinoin and an inhibition of hypertriglyceridaemia secondary to etretinate, when patients received fish oil supplementation.[107] Another pilot study showed that fish oil supplementation decreases serum triglyceride levels in psoriatic patients receiving etretinate and acitretin therapy.[108] However, in view of the small effect on increased serum cholesterol levels, cholesterol-lowering agents might be beneficial adjunctive therapy.

Teratogenicity

The potential toxicity of retinoids to the embryo is well documented. In animal experiments, vitamin A, isotretinoin, etretinate, and its main metabolite acitretin have been shown to cause various embryopathies.[109] In spite of the strict precautions recommended for women of childbearing potential, as of August 1984 a total of 214 pregnancies had occurred in women exposed to isotretinoin in the USA, with an additional 128 reported outside the USA.[110] The number of pregnancies during etretinate treatment was 24, and an additional 37 cases were reported within 2 years of discontinuation of etretinate. By November 1985, 44 cases of congenital malformation and 33 cases of spontaneous abortion had been reported in association with isotretinoin, and seven congenital defects and one stillbirth in association with etretinate.[111] The congenital malformations were craniofacial, central nervous system and cardiac abnormalities. Most common were anotia/microtia, small or absent external ear canals, hydrocephalus, cranial nerve dysfunction, septal defects, aortic arch abnormalities and thymic aplasia. Of 36 prospectively identified isotretinoin-exposed pregnancies, eight resulted in spontaneous abortion, five resulted in congenital malformations and 23 were successfully concluded without detected abnormalities.[112]

Isotretinoin-exposed pregnancies were reported to be associated with high relative risks,[68,113] for a group of selected major malformations.[112] With etretinate, the congenital malformations were craniofacial, limb and central nervous system defects. Among the 37 pregnancies occurring within 2 years of termination of treatment, three possibly etretinate-related congenital malformations were reported. Interestingly, cardiac abnormalities have not been reported with etretinate, suggesting that the pattern of abnormalities observed with the two retinoids may be different. The potential development of cognitive, emotional and behavioural abnormalities in children who do not show physical birth defects is a matter of future concern, since hypervitaminosis A in rats is associated with behavioural dysfunction.[114] It should be emphasized that several infants have been found to have evidence of central nervous system abnormalities even though they were reported to be normal at birth.[115]

The mechanism responsible for multiple congenital malformations in babies exposed to retinoids may be related to inhibition of cephalic neural crest cell activity.[116] Premigratory extirpation of part of the cephalic neural crest in chick embryos results in conotruncal heart defects and thymic malformations.[117] The fetuses of pregnant mice treated with isotretinoin show major effects on neural crest cell populations, including a spectrum of malformations resembling those reported in human infants.[112]

It has been estimated that 160 000 fertile women received isotretinoin in the first 16 months of its use in the USA,[112] whereas etretinate was mainly given to adults with psoriasis. Strict instructions and precautions are necessary for women of child-bearing potential. The administration of isotretinoin to female patients in the reproductive years is justified only in severe acne. In such cases, regular monitoring, including pregnancy tests before and after the period of treatment, is mandatory. Appropriate contraceptive measures must be used. The coincident use of oral contraceptives and isotretinoin is associated with no adverse interactions.[118]

Because of its long half-life, the use of etretinate in fertile women should be much more restricted than the use of isotretinoin. Trace levels of etretinate can be detected in the blood for up to 2 years after cessation of treatment. It therefore seems appropriate to limit its use in fertile women to those who have undergone sterilization.

No reports have yet appeared describing acitretin-induced teratogenicity in humans.

There is no evidence that retinoids are mutagens.[119] Several studies have investigated spermatogenesis in males receiving oral synthetic retinoids. In therapeutic doses, etretinate and isotretinoin do not inhibit spermatogenesis or impair the motility or morphology of sperm.[120] Indeed, increased sperm concentrations and improved motility have been observed.[121] Furthermore, fructolysis (degradation of fructose to lactate and carbon dioxide), which constitutes the main energy source in human sperm, seems unlikely to be impaired with therapeutic retinoid doses.[122] Isotretinoin treatment does not change serum levels of follicle-stimulating hormone, but does cause an insignificant decrease in serum levels of luteinizing hormone and testosterone.[123] Ellis and Voorhees have observed several men who complained of impotence during treatment with etretinate, but the relation to the drug could not be confirmed.[4] There are also reports of sexual dysfunction and menstrual changes associated with etretinate that disappear along with other more common side-effects after the drug is stopped.[124]

Topical retinoids

Both topical tretinoin and topical isotretinoin can cause a toxic dermatitis. Most patients who use tretinoin in lotion, gel or cream for acne or for photodamage experience pinkness, slight scaling and some soreness at the site of application. This 'retinoid dermatitis' is more common in blue-eyed, fair-complexioned individuals with sensitive skin. It tends to improve after continued use. Photosensitivity is a not infrequent complaint in patients using topical retinoids. Various complicated explanations for this have been suggested, but it seems most likely that it is due to the thinning of the stratum corneum that always occurs with this agent. The question of potential carcinogenicity is a contentious one – certainly as far as animal studies are concerned. There have been some studies suggesting that there is increased formation of UVR-induced tumours in mice after topical tretinoin, but an equal number showing a protective effect – as well as some showing no effect at all!

With regard to systemic toxicity from topical application, all evidence indicates that insufficient is absorbed for any significant effects.

References

1. Bartolozzi G, Bernini G, Chronic hypervitaminosis A. *Helv Paediat Acta* (1970) **15**: 301–4.
2. Bollag W, The development of retinoids in experimental and clinical oncology and dermatology. *J Am Acad Dermatol* (1983) **9**: 797–805.
3. Brunno NP, Beacham BE, Burnett JW, Adverse effects of isotretinoin therapy. *Cutis* (1984) **33**: 484–6.
4. Ellis CN, Voorhees JJ, Etretinate therapy. *J Am Acad Dermatol* (1987) **16**: 257–91.
5. Strauss JS, Rapini RP, Shalita AR et al, Isotretinoin therapy for acne: results of multicenter dose-response study. *J Am acad Dermatol* (1984) **10**: 490–6.
6. Windhorst DB, Nigra T, General clinical toxicology of oral retinoids. *J Am Acad Dermatol* (1982) **6**: 675–82.
7. Graham ML, Corey R, Califf R et al, Isotretinoin and *Staphylococcus aureus* infection. *Arch Dermatol* (1986) **122**: 815–17.
8. James WD, *Staphylococcus aureus* and etretinate. *Arch Dermatol* (1986) **122**: 976–7.
9. Elias PM, Williams ML, Retinoids, cancer and the skin. *Arch Dermatol* (1981) **117**: 160–80.
10. Molin L, Thomsen K, Wolden G et al, Retinoid dermatitis mimicking progression in mycosis fungoides: a report from Scandinavian Mycosis Fungoids Group. *Acta Derm Venereol (Stockh)* (1985) **65**: 69–71.
11. Taieb A, Maleville J, Retinoid dermatitis mimicking "eczema craquelé" *Acta Derm Venereol (Stockh)* (1985) **65**: 570
12. Levin J, Almeyda J, Erythroderma due to etretinate. *Br J Dermatol* (1985) **112**: 373–4.
13. Diffey BL, Spiro JG, Hindson TC, Photosensitivity studies and isotretinoin therapy. *J Am Acad Dermatol* (1985) **12**: 119–20.
14. Ferguson J, Johnson BE, Photosensitivity due to retinoids: clinical and laboratory studies. *Br J Dermatol* (1986) **115**: 275–83.
15. Collins MRL, James WD, Rodman VG, Etretinate photosensitivity. *J Am Acad Dermatol* (1986) **14**: 274.
16. Shalita AR, Cunningham WJ, Leyden JJ et al, Isotretinoin treatment of acne and related disorders: an update. *J Am Acad Dermatol* (1983) **9**: 629–38.
17. David M, Ginzburg A, Hodak G et al, Palmoplantar eruption associated with etretinate therapy. *Acta Derm Venereol (Stockh)* (1986) **66**: 87–9.
18. Saurat JH, Merto Y, Etretinate therapy and palmoplantar lesions (letter). *Acta Derm Venereol (Stockh)* (1986) **66**: 458.
19. Boer J, Smeenk G, Nodular prurigo-like eruption induced by etretinate. *Br J Dermatol* (1987) **116**: 271–4.
20. Crivellato E, A rosacea-like eruption induced by Tigason Ro 19-935g treatment. *Acta Derm Venereol (Stockh)* (1982) **62**: 450–2.
21. Foged EK, Jacobson FK, Side effects due to RO-9359 (Tigason): a retrospective study. *Dermatologica* (1982) **164**: 395–403.
22. Goldstein JA, Socha-SzottA, Thomsen RS et al, Comparative effect of isotretinoin and etretinate on acne and sebaceous gland secretion. *J Am Acad Dermatol* (1982) **6**: 760–5.
23. Lauharanta J, Lassus A, Combined therapy with oral retinoid and PUVA baths in severe psoriasis. *Br J Dermatol* (1981) **104**: 325.
24. Archer CB, Cerio R, Griffiths WAD, Etretinate and acquired kinking of the hair. *Br J Dermatol* (1987) **12**: 239.
25. Hayes SB, Camisa C, Acquired pili torti in two patients treated with synthetic retinoids. *Cutis* (1985) **25**: 466–8.
26. Ferguson MM, Simpson NB, Hammersley N, Severe nail dystrophy associated with retinoid therapy. *Lancet* (1983) **i**: 974.
27. Hodak E, David M, Feuerman EJ, Excessive granulation tissue during etretinate therapy. *J Am Acad Dermatol* (1984) **11**: 1166–67.
28. Chalker DK, Lesher J, Smith JG et al, Efficacy of topical isotretinoin in acne vulgaris. *J Am Acad Dermatol* (1987) **17**: 250–4.
29. Exner JH, Dahod S, Pochi PE, Pyogenic granuloma like acne lesions during isotretinoin therapy. *Arch Dermatol* (1983) **119**: 808–11.

30. Van der Rhee HJ, Combined treatment of psoriasis with a new aromatic retinoid (Tigason) in low dosage orally and triamcinolone acetonide cream topically: a double blind trial. *Br J Dermatol* (1980) **102**: 203–12.
31. Williamson DM, Greenwood R, Multiple pyogenic granulomata occurring during etretinate therapy. *Br J Dermatol* (1983) **109**: 615–19.
32. Kramer M, Excessive cerumen production due to the aromatic retinoid Tigason, in a patient with Darier's disease. *Acta Derm Venereol (Stockh)* (1982) **62**: 267–8.
33. Juhlin L, Ear ache during etretinate treatment. *Acta Derm Venereol (Stockh)* (1983) **63**: 182.
34. Rismondo V, Ubels JL, Isotretinoin in lacrimal gland fluid and tears. *Arch Ophthalmol* (1987) **105**: 416–20.
35. Kingston TP, Lowe NJ, Winston J et al, Visual and cutaneous toxicity which occurs during N-(4-hydroxyphenyl) retinamide therapy for psoriasis. *Clin Exp Dermatol* (1986) **11**: 624–7.
36. Fraunfelder FT, Labraico JM, Meyer M, Adverse ocular reactions possibly associated with isotretinoin. *Am J Ophthalmol* (1985) **100**: 534–7.
37. Milson J, Jones PH, King K et al, Ophthalmological effects of 13-*cis*-retinoic acid therapy for acne vulgaris. *Br J Dermatol* (1981) **107**: 491.
38. Bluckman HS, Peck GL, Olsen TG et al, Blepharoconjunctivitis: a side effect of 13-*cis*-retinoic acid therapy for dermatologic disease. *Ophthalmology* (1979) **86**: 753–8.
39. Weleber RG, Denman ST, Hanifin JM et al, Abnormal retinal function associated with isotretinoin therapy for acne. *Arch Ophthalmol* (1986) **104**: 831–7.
40. Grattan CEH, Brown RD, Cowan MA et al, Retinoids and eye-reduced function with isotretinoin. *Br J Dermatol* (1987) **117** (suppl 32): 23.
41. Kaiser-Kupfer MI, Peck GL, Carusa RL et al, Abnormal retinal function associated with fenretinide: a synthetic retinoid. *Arch Ophthalmol* (1986) **104**: 69–70.
42. Palastine AG, Transient acute myopia resulting from isotretinoin (Accutane) therapy. *Am Ophthalmol* (1984) **16**: 660–2.
43. Watson NJ, Hutchinson CH, Rod and cone malfunction as a manifestation of isotretinoin therapy – a case report. *J Dermatol Treat* (1992) **3**: 205–7.
44. Dicken CH, Retinoids: a review. *J Am Acad Dermatol* (1984) **11**: 541–52.
45. McBurney EI, Rosen DA, Elevated cretin phosphokinase with isotretinoin. *J Am Acad Dermatol* (1983) **10**: 528–9.
46. Chen D, Rofksy HE, Elevated CPK and isotretinoin. *J Am Acad Dermatol* (1985) **12**: 582–3.
47. Hodak E, Godath N, David M et al, Muscle damage induced by isotretinoin. *Br Med J* (1986) **293**: 425–6.
48. Jacyk WK, Elevated creatine phosphokinase levels associated with the use of etretinate. *J Am Acad Dermatol* (1986) **15**: 710.
49. Ellis CN, Gilbert M, Cohen KA et al, Increased muscle tone during etretinate therapy. *J Am Acad Dermatol* (1986) **14**: 907–9.
50. Hodak E, David M, Gadoth N et al, Etretinate-induced muscle damage. *Br J Dermatol* (1987) **116**: 623–6.
51. Korner W, Vollin Y, New aspects of the tolerance of retinol in humans. *Int J Vitam Nutr Res* (1972) **45**: 363–72.
52. Ruby LK, Mohinder AM, Skeletal deformities following chronic hypervitaminosis A. *J Bone Joint Surg [Am]* (1974) **56**: 1283–7.
53. Prendiville J, Bingham EA, Burrows D, Premature epiphyseal closure – a complication of etretinate therapy in children. *J Am Acad Dermatol* (1986) **15**: 1259–62.
54. Tamayo L, Ruiz-Maldonado R, Oral retinoid (ro-10-9359) in children with lamellar ichthyosis, epidermolytic hyperkeratosis and symmetrical progressive erythrokeratoderma. *Dermatologica* (1980) **161**: 305–14.
55. Tamayo L, Ruiz-Maldonado R, Long term follow-up of 30 children under oral retinoid (RO 10-9359). In: Orfanos CE, Cunningham WJ, Leyden JJ et al (eds). *Retinoids: advances in basic research and therapy.* Springer: Berlin, 1981, pp 287–94.
56. DiGiovanna JJ, Peck GL, Oral synthetic retinoid treatment in children. *Pediat Dermatol* (1983) **1**: 177–88.
57. Brun P, Baran R, Neonatal ichthyosis treated for seven years with etretinate without side

effects on growth or ossification: a case report. *Curr Ther Res* (1986) **40**: 657–63.

58. Glover MT, Peters AM, Atherdon DJ, Surveillance for skeletal toxicity of children treated with etretinate. *Br J Dermatol* (1987) **116**: 609–14.
59. Mills CM, McGuire J, Aslow RC, Premature epiphyseal closure in a child receiving oral 13-*cis*-retinoic acid. *Drug Safety* (1993) **9**: 280–290.
60. Milstone LM, McGuire J, Aslow RC, Premature epiphyseal closure in a child receiving oral 13-*cis*-retinoic acid. *J Am Acad Dermatol* (1982) **7**: 633–66.
61. McGuire J, Milstone L, Lawston J, Isotretinoin administration alters juvenile and adult bone. In: Saurat J (ed.). *Retinoids: new trends in research and therapy*. Karger: Basel, 1985, pp 419–39.
62. Pittsley RA, Yuoder FW, Retinoid hyperostosis skeletal toxicity associated with long-term administration of 13-*cis*-retinoic acid for refractory ichthyosis. *N Engl J Med* (1983) **308**: 1012–4.
63. Gerber LH, Helfgott RK, Gross GG et al, Vertebral abnormalities associated with synthetic retinoid use. *J Am Acad Dermatol* (1984) **10**: 817–23.
64. Ellis CN, Madison KC, Pennes DR et al, Isotretinoin therapy is associated with early skeletal radiographic changes. *J Am Acad Dermatol* (1984) **10**: 1024–9.
65. Ellis CN, Pennes DR, Madison KC et al, Skeletal radiographic changes during retinoid therapy. In: Saurat J (ed.). *Retinoids: new trends in research and therapy*. Karger: Basel, 1985, pp 440–4.
66. Gross E, Helfgott R, Hicks J et al, Evaluation of vertebral spine osteoporosis in patients treated with isotretinoin. *Clin Res* (1985) **33**: 642.
67. Kilcoyne RF, Cope R, Cunningham W et al, Minimal spinal hyperostosis with low-dose isotretinoin therapy. *Invest Radiol* (1986) **21**: 41–4.
68. DiGiovanna JJ, Helfgott R, Gerber GL et al, Extraspinal tendon and ligament calcification after long-term isotretinoin therapy (abstract). *J Invest Dermatol* (1987) **88**: 485.
69. Gilbert M, Ellis CN, Voorhees JJ, Lack of skeletal radiographic changes during short-term etretinate therapy for psoriasis. *Dermatologica* (1986) **192**: 160–3.
70. Burge S, Ryan T, Diffuse hyperostosis associated with etretinate. *Lancet* (1985) **ii**: 397–8.
71. Sillevis Smith JH, De Mari FE, A serious side effect of etretinate (Tigason). *Clin Exp Dermatol* (1984) **9**: 554–6.
72. DeGiovanna JJ, Helfgott RK, Gerber LH et al, Extraspinal tendon and ligament calcification associated with long-term therapy with etretinate. *N Engl J Med* (1986) **315**: 1177-82.
73. Simpson KR, Rosenbach A, Lowe NJ, Etretinate for retinoid-responsive dermatoses: further observations of long-term therapy. *J Dermatol Treat* (1993) **4**: 179–82.
74. Tfelt-Hausen P, Knudsen B, Peterson F et al, Spinal cord compression after long-term etretinate. *Lancet* (1989) **ii**: 325–6.
75. Zabarius P, Krause E, Gay-Bobo A et al, Ossification de la membrane inter-osseuse antibrachiale sous etretinate. *Am Dermatol Venereol* (1989) **116**: 123–6.
76. Margolis D, Attie M, Leyden JJ, Effects of isotretinoin on bone demineralization. *Arch Dermatol* (1996) **132**: 769–74.
77. Lawson JP, Maguire J, The spectrum of skeletal changes associated with long term administration of 13-*cis*-retinoic acid. *Skeletal Radiol* (1987) **16**: 91–7.
78. Viraben R, Mathien C, Fontan B, Benign intracranial hypertension during etretinate therapy for mycosis fungoides. *J Am Acad Dermatol* (1985) **12**: 515–17.
79. Lindemayer H, Isotretinoin intoxication in attempted suicide. *Acda Derm Venereol (Stockh)* (1986) **66**: 452–3.
80. Hazen PG, Carney JF, Walker AE et al, Depression – a side effect of 13-cis retinoic acid therapy. *J Am Acad Dermatol* (1983) **8**: 278–9.
81. Helfman RJ, Brickman M, Fahey J, Isotretinoin dermatitis simulating acute pityriasis rosea. *Cutis* (1984) **33**: 297–300.
82. Weiss VC, Layden T, Spinowitz A et al, Chronic active hepatitis associated with etretinate therapy. *Br J Dermatol* (1985) **112**: 591–7.
83. Weiss VC, West DD, Ackerman R et al, Hepatotoxic reactions in patient treated with etretinate. *Arch Dermatol* (1984) **120**: 104–6.
84. Fontan B, Bonafe JL, Moatti JP, Toxic effect of the aromatic retinoid etretinate. *Arch Dermatol* (1983) **119**: 187–8.

85. Rubin MG, Hanno R, Short term etretinate for pustular psoriasis. *J Am Acad Dermatol* (1985) **12**: 896–7.
86. Hoffmann La Roche, *Tegison information brochure*. Nutley: New Jersey, April 1987.
87. Van Voorst PC, Houthoff HJ, Eggink HF et al, Etretinate (Tigason) hepatitis in 2 patients. *Dermatologica* (1984) **168**: 41–6.
88. Wong RC, Gilbert M, Yoo TY et al, Photosensitivity and isotretinoin therapy. *J Am Acad Dermatol* (1986) **14**: 1095–6.
89. Vahlquist A, Loof L, Mordlinder H et al, Differential hepatoxicity of two oral retinoids (etretinate and isotretinoin) in a patient with palmo plantar psoriasis. *Acta Derm Venereol (Stockh)* (1985) **65**: 359–62.
90. Zachariae H, Roged E, Bjerring P et al, Liver biopsy during etretinate (Tigason) treatment. In: Saurat J (ed.). *Retinoids: new trends in research and therapy*. Karger: Basel, 1985, pp 494–7.
91. Van Voorst PC, Houthoff HJ, Gips CH et al, Hepatologic side effects during long-term retinoid therapy: to cells and portal hypertension. In: Saurat J (ed.). *Retinoids: new trends in research and therapy*. Karger: Basel, 1985, pp 498–500.
92. Roenigk HH Jr, Retinoids: effect on the liver. In: Saurat J (ed.). *Retinoids: new trends in research and therapy*. Karger: Basel, 1985, pp 476–88.
93. Camuto P, Shupack J, Orbuch P et al, Long term effects of etretinate on the liver in psoriasis. *Am J Surg Pathol* (1987) **11**: 30–7.
94. Kingston TP, Matt L, Lowe NJ, Etretin therapy for severe psoriasis. *Arch Dermatol* (1987) **123**: 55–8.
95. Lassus A, Geiger JM, Nyblom M et al, Treatment of severe psoriasis with etretin (Ro 10-1670). *Br J Dermatol* (1987) **117**: 333–41.
96. Lyons F, Laker MF, Marsden JR et al, Effect of oral 13-*cis*-retinoic acid on serum lipids. *Br J Dermatol* (1982) **107**: 591.
97. Vahlquist C, Michaelsson G, Valquist A et al, A sequential comparison of etretinate and isotretinoin proteins. *Br J Dermatol* (1985) **112**: 69–76.
98. Gollnick H, Schwartzkopf W, Proschle W et al, Retinoid and blood lipids: an update and review. In: Saurat J (ed.). *Retinoids: new trends in research and therapy*. Karger: Basel, 1985, p 445.
99. Zech LA, Gross EG, McClean SW et al, Lipoprotein metabolism in patients receiving synthetic retinoids isotretinoin and etretinate. *Arteriosclerosis* (1987) **1**: 39A.
100. Ellis CN, Swanson NA, Grekin RC et al, Etretinate therapy causes increases in lipid levels in patients with psoriasis. *Arch Dermatol* (1982) **8**: 559–62.
101. Marsden JR, Laker MF, Shuster S, Biochemical effects of isotretinoin. In: Saurat J (ed.). *Retinoids: new trends in research and therapy*. Karger: Basel, 1985, p 461.
102. Merot Y, Camenzind M, Geisen J et al, Arotinoid ethyl ester (RO 13-6298): a long term pilot study in various dermatoses. *Acta Derm Venereol (Stockh)* (1987) **67**: 237–42.
103. Marsden J, Hyperlipidemia due to isotretinoin and etretinate: possible mechanisms and consequences. *Br J Dermatol* (1986) **114**: 401–2.
104. Laker MF, Green C, Bhuiyan AKMJ et al, Isotretinoin and serum lipids: studies on fatty acid, apoprotein and intermediary metabolism. *Br J Dermatol* (1987) **117**: 203–6.
105. Dicken CH, Connoly SM, Eruptive xanthoma associated with isotretinoin. *Arch Dermatol* (1980) **116**: 951–2.
106. Bershad G, Rubinstein A, Patterniti JR et al, Changes in plasma lipids and lipoprotein during isotretinoin therapy for acne. *N Engl J Med* (1985) **313**: 981–5.
107. Marsden JR, Effect of dietary fish oil on hyperlipidemia due to isotretinoin and etretinate. *Hum Toxicol* (1987) **6**: 219–22.
108. Lowe N, Ashley J, Borok M et al, Fish oil supplementation causes decreases in serum triglyceride levels (letter). *Arch Dermatol* (1988) **124**: 177.
109. Geelen JAG, Hypervitaminosis A-induced teratogenesis. *CRC Crit Rev Toxicol* (1979) **6**: 351–75.
110. Chen DT, Human pregnancy experience with the retinoids. In: Saurat J (ed.). *Retinoids: new trends in research and therapy*. Karger: Basel, 1985, pp 398–406.
111. Rosa FW, Wilk AL, Kelsey FO, Teratogen update: vitamin A congeners. *Teratology* (1986) **33**: 355–64.

112. Lammer EJ, Chen DT, Hoar RM et al, Retinoic acid embryopathy. *N Engl J Med* (1985) **313**: 837–41.
113. Bollag W, Arotinoids: a new class of retinoid with activities in oncology and dermatology. *Cancer Chemother Pharmacol* (1981) **7**: 27–9.
114. Voorhees CV, Retinoic acid embryopathy (letter). *N Engl J Med* (1986) **315**: 262–3.
115. Hersh JH, Danhauer DS, Hand ME et al, Retinoic acid embryopathy: timing of exposure and effects on fetal development. *J Am Med Assoc* (1985) **254**: 900–10.
116. Benke PJ, The isotretinoin teratogen syndrome. *J Am Med Assoc* (1984) **251**: 3267–9.
117. Kirby ML, Gale TF, Stewart DE, Neural crest cells contribute to normal aorticopulmonary separation. *Science* (1983) **220**: 1056–61.
118. Orme M, Back DJ, Shaw MH et al, Isotretinoin and contraception. *Lancet* (1984) **ii**: 752–3.
119. Kamm JJ, Ashenfelter KO, Ehmann CW, Preclinical and clinical toxicology of selected retinoids. In: Sporn B, Roberts AB, Dewitt S et al (eds). *The retinoids*, Vol 2. Academic Press: Orlando, 1984, pp 287–326.
120. Schill WB, Wagner A, Nikolowsky J et al, Aromatic retinoid and 13-*cis*-retinoic acid: spermatological investigation. In: Orfanos CE, Braun-Talco J, Farber GM et al (eds). *Retinoids: advances in basic research and therapy*. Springer: Berlin, 1981, pp 389–99.
121. Torok L, Spermatological examinations in males treated with etretinate. In: Cunliffe WJ, Miller AJ (eds). *Retinoid therapy*. MTP Press: Lancaster, 1984, pp 161–4.
122. Lauharanta J, Kapyaho K, Kanerva L, Effect of retinoids on the fructolytic activity of human spermatoza. In: Saurat J (ed.). *Retinoids: new trends in research and therapy*. Karger: Basel, 1985, pp 411–14.
123. Torok L, Kasa M, Spermatological and endocrinological examinations connected with isotretinoin treatment. In: Saurat J (ed.). *Retinoids: new trends in research and therapy*. Karger: Basel, 1985, pp 407–41.
124. Halker-Sorenson L, Menstrual changes in a patient treated with etretinate. *Lancet* (1987) **ii**: 636.

Index

Abbreviations used; CRABP, Cytosolic (cellular) retinoic acid-binding protein; RAR, Retinoic acid receptor; RXR, Retinoid X receptor